Praise for *Misdiagnosed*:

"... Jean's story defines **resiliency**.... Her lack of resentment for having to spend three decades in a body that won't work will simply **amaze the reader**. In a word, Jean is grace personified."

—Cregg K., Milwaukee, WI

"Jean's story is truly **inspirational**. Reading her memoir has reminded me to appreciate the simple things in life. From page to page, my emotions would shift. One moment, a tear would stream down my face as she described her experiences living with a disability as a child. Then, the next moment I would giggle and think to myself, "I can *totally* relate to that".... Jean reminds us that **living with a disability is an adversity, but not a road block**."

—Angela P., Plymouth, MN

"... I couldn't put [*Misdiagnosed*] down! From the very beginning it was clear that her **positive attitude** was something ingrained in her DNA.... Jean's book had me laughing one minute and then anxious to see what came next.... **A wonderful, inspiring book for anyone struggling with a medical diagnosis** or simply struggling to remember the positives in their life."

— Leann N., Minnetonka, MN

"I appreciate the **honest** accounts of her story.... **Best book** I have read in a long time."

—Tammy A., Winona, MN

MISDIAGNOSED

Misdiagnosed

My Thirty-Year Struggle with a Debilitating Disorder I Never Had

Jean Sharon Abbott

JSA

Published by Jean Sharon Abbott

Publisher's Cataloging-In-Publication Data
(Prepared by The Donohue Group, Inc.)

Abbott, Jean Sharon.

    Misdiagnosed : my thirty-year struggle with a debilitating disorder I never had / Jean Sharon Abbott.

      pages :   illustrations ;   cm

    Issued also as an ebook.

    ISBN: 978-0-9969793-0-6

    1. Abbott, Jean Sharon—Health. 2. Dystonia—Patients—Biography. 3. Movement disorders—Patients—Biography. 4. Cerebral palsied—Biography. 5. Diagnostic errors. I. Title.

RC935.D8 .A22 2015

                           616.74/092

Design and Production by Mighty Media, Inc.
Cover: Kelly Doudna · Interior: Chris Long

Personal and family photographs supplied by the author; back cover photograph supplied by Jason Narverud Photography

Printed in the United States of America
First Printing 2015

ISBN 978-0-9969793-0-6

JeanAbbott.com

Dedicated to

MOM AND DAD . . .

thank you for raising me to be a strong and positive woman. Not once did I feel like a burden, and you taught me that I can do anything. I thank God every night that He chose you to be my parents.

STEVE, MY BEST FRIEND . . .

one of my greatest gifts in life was that you were able to see past my physical limitations and love me for me. You've seen me at my strongest and you've seen me at my weakest, yet you never stopped loving me.

MY CHILDREN, WINONA, SHARON, AND JOHN . . .

thank you for understanding all the times I had to stop playing with you to work on this book. I hope that you've learned that you can make any dreams come true as long as you're willing to put in the work. I thank God for choosing me to be your mom, a gift I never thought possible.

Contents

Acknowledgments

THERE ARE CERTAIN PEOPLE THAT I HAVE TO THANK. WITH-
out their support during this project (and throughout my life), this
book would not be possible.

Jan Pavloski, who assisted me in editing and organizing this
manuscript. Without you, it would still be a draft on my computer.
Nancy Dumke, who encouraged me to bring this book to comple-
tion, and introduced me to Jan. Penny Steele, for introducing me
to Mark Brokering, who educated me about the publishing process
and creating this wonderful title. The staff at Mighty Media: Nancy
Tuminelly, Pam Chenevert, and Lauren Kukla, who helped me get
this project across the finish line.

My family, especially my brothers. You never treated me like a
fragile dish, which prepared me for the world! My nieces and nephews (Mikaela, Sophia, Rebecca, Jack, Samantha, and Henry) for your
never-ending encouragement and thinking BIG! I agree; we need to
make this into a movie! Cathy and Michelle, we may not be sisters
by blood, but you have both helped me out in ways that I can never
repay. And, of course, Steve's family. I am so lucky to have you all in
my life.

My friends ... there are far too many to mention by name. For
those of you who have been by my side since I was a young girl, I
thank you for the laughs. Even more so, I thank you for standing
by my side when it would have been easier to walk away. And to
my new friends, who never got to know the "old" me but can still
appreciate why I have so much to give thanks for.

Last, but not least, God. Even as young child, I knew you made me "different" for a reason. I may not have understood why, and may have questioned your decision at times, but I accepted it, knowing that God doesn't make mistakes. I thank you for giving me a physically challenging life. I now have a better appreciation for the little things and have been blessed to share my amazing journey with the world, in turn helping to change the lives of others in a positive way.

Introduction

IF YOU HAVE A PULSE, YOU KNOW INJUSTICE WHEN YOU HEAR it. A twelve-year-old girl subjected to—some might say mutilated by—a doctor's scalpel; poked and prodded with needles, humiliated by cold, invasive procedures—hopeless tests ... for what purpose? To validate one doctor's reputation as an "expert" in the field of pediatric neurology? To pad the ego of a man with whom every hospital consulted—even the world-renowned clinic I visited for a week? Because no one else in the medical world bothered to seek advances in a physical disability found among anonymous children ... children who should be thankful that someone with a medical degree cared to take on a patient who would never improve?

This could have been my attitude. This could have been my family's tone throughout my blogging adventures on *Rainy Day Friend...The Journey from Wheels to Heels*, and throughout my life. This could be a book about anger, resentment, regrets, and evening scores. But it isn't. It's quite the opposite. Why? Because I had a choice. Because my family and I chose resilience over anger, acceptance instead of lawsuits.

Sure, my book is a story about unnecessary struggle. I was misdiagnosed! I was missing the cure. For most of my life, I could have been swallowing a little pill that would have allowed me to rollerskate, allure a prom date, and perhaps pursue sports like my friends. But instead it's a story of endurance, acquiescence, forgiveness—and always, always, always moving forward. It's a book about discovery. And, finally, it's a journey out of suffering to a state of gratitude that can only be felt by those who stumble through it with me, step by awkward—and sometimes painful—step.

It's a bit of an out-of-body experience to tell this little girl's tale of hospital stays and medical procedures. Yet that was me ... and for three decades whenever I heard, "Can I ask you a question?" the words, "I have spastic diplegia," shot out of my mouth faster than most can order a cheeseburger from McDonald's. This neurological muscle disorder is very similar to cerebral palsy. Many people would ask if I had CP, and for years I didn't even know what that was.

Growing up with spastic diplegia as my label, muscle spasticity limited my everyday tasks. Walking home from the bus stop at the end of a long school day challenged me, even before the Minnesota snow flew. My knees would knock, and I'd literally trip myself, stumbling—sometimes falling for the whole neighborhood to see. Eternally on my tippy-toes, I was like a ballerina, but without the grace. My left arm tightened up like a frozen chicken wing strapped to my side. Once home, schoolwork consumed the rest of the night, since holding a pencil was an arduous task. Writing homework responses so my teachers could read them was daily torture for a little girl whose mind worked far faster than her body parts.

When my friends and I got together, we'd play Barbies and board games for hours, making me the perfect bad-weather friend. Of course, on sunny days, I tried to run around outside, but after a while I would tire. We'd make our way to the garage where my kittens were, but eventually we'd head back inside for another Barbie marathon.

Some time ago, I told my mom that I wanted to write a book, but I had no idea what title to give it. Without hesitation, she told me this: "When you were a little girl, I thought that if a book was written about you, it should be called *Rainy Day Friend*."

I looked at her and asked, "Why?"

"When you were little, your friends wouldn't call to see if you could play on the sunny days. But when it rained, you had many playdate requests. You were the perfect rainy day friend."

I find it really important to add that while growing up I had wonderful friends. I don't know if it's possible to have found better friendships in my life. They didn't care that it took me longer than the other kids to do things ... and if they did, they never let on about it. These girls helped to make me the person I am today. In fact, they are still my best friends ... the people I love to laugh with, and trust with my deepest thoughts.

From time to time, I would let my spasticity get the best of me and yell to my mom, "Other people just do things!" I'd watch my peers race around the playground or walk with poise to class. I couldn't help but wonder, *How do they do that?*

Yet with great parents, lots of friends, and a growing faith, I was able to live a "normal" life. I wasn't about to let my inabilities stop me from having fun. People would always comment on how positive I was, even though there were so many things I couldn't do. I was just living—the only way I knew how. I had all the same dreams that non-disabled girls had: moving away to college, finding the perfect man to marry, having kids and raising them to be happy and hopeful—like me!

I lived much of my life finding my dreams challenged on a daily basis. I believed I had a debilitating disorder which could only get worse with time. Then, just when I didn't believe it could get any darker, a miracle happened—an amazing gift changed my struggle and altered my journey forever.

For so many reasons, I know I must use this precious gift of mobility to the fullest. Many people experience life-changing events that are a 180 from my new diagnosis ... the death of a spouse or child, spine-crippling accidents, devastating diagnoses like ALS or cancer. I owe them, and all who battled with me through the darkest days, a debt of gratitude I cannot begin to repay. My struggle has ended ... my prayers were answered. How could I be anything but grateful?

Although I've had a good life, the many obstacles I faced often make my story sad. Yet, I loved my childhood ... with its highlights to make up for the hard times. And at the darkest points, I had a support system that I wouldn't trade for the world. Here's my struggle— here's my story. Don't feel sorry for me. Even if I had the chance, I wouldn't change a thing.

Crooked Legs, Crowded Room

EVERYTHING IS BRIGHT YET BLURRY. THE BED I'M LYING ON is moving at a gentle pace down the hall. The nurse dressed in baby blue scrubs looks down at me with an empathetic smile. *It's over*, I think to myself.

"We're going to bring you to your room," the nurse says sweetly. "You're doing a great job," she says as the bed turns the corner and squeezes through the double doors. In my mind, I nod my head. However, I know I'm so exhausted my head's not budging.

The nurses drive my gurney up to a standard hospital bed—my home for the next three days. "On the count of three," one says. The sheets lift me, a nurse on each end. Pain pierces through my legs from one side of my body to the other. I want to cry out and scream, but I know that it will do no good. Instead, I let two little tears from my twelve-year-old eyes drip down the sides of my cheeks. Silently, I pray for my parents' arrival. I'm relieved when I see them round the corner and enter my room. I know that everything will be okay now that they are by my side.

I can see in my father's eyes that he wishes it were him in the bed and not me. My mom rubs my arm. Her smile assures me that the worst is over. That's when it hits me. *I'm in a body cast.*

I place my hands on my stomach and feel the hard, rough plaster shell that will force me to stay still while my muscles heal correctly. I remember the doctors saying that the cast would go from my rib cage down to my knees. They didn't lie. I will spend the next three weeks in a bed unable to move. I'm petrified. *Does the pain come with*

1

the cast? Will it hurt this badly for the next month? And then the muscle spasms begin.

"It hurts so much," I tell my parents. Every time my muscles clench, pain and fear seize my body. The greater the pain, the more my muscles tighten up. *This has to stop and soon, because there is no way that I can get through this.*

My dad wets a white washcloth from the hospital bathroom and returns to my right side. He sits in a chair, and with the washcloth, he gently rubs my head. He moves the cool cloth from the bottom portion of my forehead to my hairline. His touch is gentle and soothing. "Shhh," he says. Slowly, the spasms decline and so does the pain.

My mom's been talking with the nurse ... I'm not sure why. Then the nurse leaves for a moment and returns just as fast. "This will help with the spasms," the nurse says, attaching a clear bag to the tall metal stand that resembles a coat rack. "This time it's Valium," she explains. I get the impression this isn't the first stuff she's put through my IV. "It will calm her muscles down, which will also help ease the pain." I'm not clear on anything said after that. All I know is that she can do whatever she wants as long as it stops the pain.

My father continues to rub my forehead even after I quit complaining. I think he's not sure what else he can do, so he does what already has worked. I'm so thankful he's by my side. Usually it's Mom who takes care of me when I am ill or have fallen and hurt myself. This is a side of Dad I don't see often.

With a little relief, I look around the room. I quickly realize that there are other patients here. I see three metal baby cribs. One infant is crying and I can hear the mother trying to comfort her. As soon as this baby calms down, another starts wailing. There is always a baby crying. I can't relax. My muscles tense up and the pain pulses through me again. These babies have to stop bawling or my pain will never cease. I know that they are just infants, but I want them gone.

I tell my mom, "Every time I hear crying, my muscles start spazzing." I can see the concern on her face and she knows that she needs to do something. As soon as another nurse comes into the room,

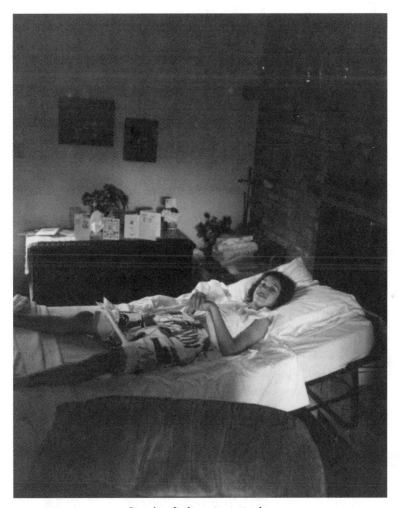

Jean in a body cast, age twelve

Mom confronts her. I imagine she's going to insist that this room simply won't work, but I know my mom better than that. She is going to be polite. I also know that she is not going to let this problem be. The nurse listens to whatever my mother has told her and then leaves the room.

The nurse returns. Now both of my parents walk over to her. I can tell they are talking. The nurse informs them of another room where they can move me. "It doesn't have young children," the nurse states in a low tone. "However, the other patient in that room is a twelve-year-old boy."

I don't want to go to a room with a boy in it! On the other hand, I can't take listening to these babies. As it turns out, I don't have any say in the decision. I will be staying in the room with the screaming babies.

I overhear the nurse tell my parents, "The youngsters in this room have had either brain or heart surgery. They are in a lot of pain, but we will do our best to keep your daughter as comfortable as possible." These kids are in much more serious condition than I am. They are little babies—they can't even tell their moms or dads how much it hurts. *Dear Lord, help me be strong so I get through this. I can deal with this, but help me to understand why these little children need to be in so much pain. I know that it will be okay, but do they?* The Valium must have kicked in—I suddenly fall asleep.

I'm not quite sure how long I slept. It must have been quite a while because my parents are getting ready to leave. I understand that they need to go home to my brothers, but I really wish that they would stay with me. I never was a big fan of sleepovers and this is hardly a slumber party. I would give anything for my mom to stay, although I don't say a word about how I feel. It would only make it harder on her. She doesn't like this situation any more than I do. So, I let them hug me and tell me goodnight. "Bye," I whisper. And then they are gone.

For the first time, I really give the room a good look. Directly to the right of me is a toddler in a crib. The little girl has a white bandage on her head, but I can still see that she is a cutie. I look to the far right wall and see the big door that goes out to the hallway. There's nothing too out of the ordinary about it. It's just extra wide. *I guess that's how they pushed me through on the riding bed.*

My view is limited. It's hard to see the entire room because my cast forces me to lie flat, yet I see the other two cribs. To my left is a big window, but the metal blinds are closed. It feels like I should be going to sleep, but I've never stayed overnight in a hospital before.

And I've never shared a room in my life. I really have no idea what to expect.

The nurse comes in and asks me if I'd like to watch some television. She takes the remote that is attached to my bed and turns it on for me. The TV is mounted from the ceiling near the foot of my bed. With all of the commotion, I hadn't noticed it. The show that is on is like none that I have ever seen before.

On the monitor, a middle-aged woman begins talking dramatically. "Tomorrow morning we will be having French toast with warm maple syrup for breakfast, boys and girls." She sounds like she just hopped out of a fairy tale. "You will also get your choice of juice," she continues, her big brown eyes growing wide with excitement. I'm not sure what to make of this. I feel as if someone has placed me in a children's television show.

"Tomorrow will be show-and-tell," she goes on. "I hope all of you have something that you can give to your nurse for just a short while, because Sam will put it on television for the whole hospital to see."

This is kinda cool, I think to myself. *This place might not be so bad after all. The nurses are nice and the people on the television are just balls of happiness.* I'll have to figure out something to give my nurse tomorrow ... just to see how nutty the guy gets when he shows it on TV.

The hospital program continues for just a little while longer and I'm beginning to get tired again. Little did I know that the room lights had been growing dimmer as I watched the lady on TV. My nurse comes in, fluffs my pillow a bit, then leaves after I tell her I'm fine. I am relieved that I don't need anything, because I think I would have been too afraid to ask for it.

The room seems too bright to go to sleep. The door to the hallway is open, and the streetlights shine in through the closed blinds, sending a stream of light down the center of our room. I lie on my back, close my eyes, and drift to sleep.

I awaken in the middle of the night to something squeezing my right arm. I slowly open my eyes and look up to see the nurse taking my blood pressure and pulse. "We need to roll you onto your side now," she says quietly not to wake the other children.

"No, I don't want to lie on my side. I want to stay on my back," I plead. My body hasn't moved an inch since they put me in this bed. I know that no matter how gentle she is when she adjusts me, the pain is going to rush through me like fire.

"You've been in the same position for several hours, honey. If I don't put you on your side, you will get bed sores," she says, trying to convince me.

"I don't want to move. I'm fine just the way I am." For the moment it doesn't hurt, and I'm petrified that the second she touches my fragile body, the pain and spasms will start all over again. I know deep down inside that "what I think" doesn't matter—she has to move me.

Another nurse comes into the room and I see now that this is going to be a two-person job. "We're going to move the sheet you're on, all the way to the right side of your bed," she explains to me. "Then we will gently roll you onto your left side."

Please just do this fast, I pray.

I feel myself move with a quick and sudden jolt. *Oh, my God!* The pain is unbearable. It feels like they just ripped the muscles off my leg bones. This is going to hurt forever. *Why did they do this to me? I shouldn't be here. This is a living nightmare.*

"Halfway there," the nurse tells me.

She's got to be kidding me. There's more? Oh, yeah … I'm still on my back, but at least the pain went away just as quickly as it came. There are nurses on both sides of my bed. The nurse on my left holds my right shoulder, while the other nurse puts her hands on my cast. Very slowly they roll me onto my left side. The pain surges through me for a brief moment.

While one nurse holds me on my side, the other nurse stuffs white pillows between my back and the side rails of the bed. For the first time since I came out of surgery, I take a real good look at my body. I am trapped in this cast, which goes from my rib cage down to just above my kneecaps. A ruler-sized bar made out of casting material separates my legs just above the knees. Because I am on my side, the bar is forcing my right leg to hang up in the air. I feel like a human triangle. I look like I got stuck doing side leg-lifts.

The nurse quickly grabs two more fluffy pillows from the cabinet next to my bed and stuffs them between my legs for extra support. Apparently, that's not enough, because she grabs one more pillow and squeezes it in the little space that remains between my top leg and the leg pillows already put in position.

"Are you comfortable?" she asks.

I nod yes, but I'm thinking, *How on God's green earth am I going to be able to sleep on my side with one leg hanging up in the air?* It's better than pain, however, so I'll take it. To my surprise I fall back to sleep just as soon as the nurses leave the room.

In the morning, I wake up to my special French toast. The nurses must have moved me again because, when I open my eyes, I am on my back. I see flower arrangements, probably from family and friends. My favorite display looks just like an ice cream sundae. It has big white carnations as the vanilla ice cream and a closed baby red rose to represent a cherry, placed perfectly in a glass sundae dish. I've never seen anything like this before. It's the perfect gift to put a smile on my face this morning. A nurse puts the flowers and cards on a shelf right in front of the window. My little area looks so cheery now.

The mom of the little girl in the crib right next to me comes into the room and hands me a *Teen Bop* magazine. "You're being such a great sport. I had to get you something."

"Thank you," I reply.

She talks to me a little bit more about the hospital staff being so nice and that her daughter has been here a few days. I can tell by the circles under her eyes that she hasn't had much sleep. She looks very concerned for the well-being of her child.

I page through the magazine just as my parents enter the room. "Good morning," they say to me.

"Where did you get the magazine?" my mom asks.

"Her," I nod my head in the direction of the woman at the crib next to me.

"Look at these flowers," Mom says as she walks over to the window.

"They're from Doug and Maryanne," I tell my parents. "It looks just like an ice cream sundae!"

Just then, another flower delivery comes in for me. It's the biggest flower arrangement that I have ever seen. It's a huge pot of purple azaleas. As Mom is reading the card, the nurse comes into the room.

"Wow! Who gave her those flowers? You?" the nurse asks my parents.

"No," my mom says surprisingly. "They're from her orthodontist."

"Must be some orthodontist," says the nurse.

The nurse turns to me and asks if I want to send something up for the show-and-tell program. I don't know what to do. I am thinking that I'm too old for this kind of stuff, but my mom suggests that I send up the flowers that look like ice cream. Being the compliant kid that I am, I go along with it.

The three days in the hospital speed by in a blur. I only recall bits and pieces, with the exception of the first time I had to pee. I came to realize that it was not going to be an easy task. It's not natural for the human body to release bodily fluids through a hole in a cast while balancing on an uncomfortable bedpan. I had the urgency to pee like no other time in my life, but my body could not relax.

My dad walked into the bathroom, just a few steps from my bed, and turned on the water in the sink. We all knew the water trick. My mom and grandma stood by my side as I tried to pee. Nothing. My dad turned on the shower making it sound like a river was getting hit with a nice downpour of rain. Nothing. *I've got to pee, but it's impossible.* My parents know that if I don't urinate soon, I will need to have a catheter. I don't know what that is, but it must not be good because now my father is flushing the toilet … one flush after another, as he runs water steadily in the sink and shower. "Ann, is she peeing now?" he yells from the other room.

The sound of Niagara Falls fills the hospital room. My grandma yells, "Roger, stop flushing the toilet!" She is clearly embarrassed.

My father continues to flush the toilet with no break. I laugh uncontrollably and I pee. *Thank God.* My mom and grandma smile to one another and announce to my father that he has succeeded.

This was my bathroom routine during the weeks I recovered from my muscle transfer surgery. Making myself laugh in order to pee was probably not the best solution to a stubborn bladder problem, and would in fact cause serious embarrassment down the road. But on this day, it was my ticket out of the hospital … my medical trick to a swift discharge. And I wanted nothing more than to go home.

Graduation Day

RECLINED ON THE ELEVATED TABLE, I RECALLED HOW PHILLIP lifted my little leg high into the air. Like an injured football player, sidelined flat on my back, I loved the burning sensation up the hamstring as the physical therapist relaxed, yet worked, my muscles. This was a stretch that my mom had executed for me all those years before I went to bed—but Phillip did it best.

On this warm spring morning, I got the kids off to school and I was on my way to see my latest physical therapist. Phillip was out of the picture by now … but the routine was not. PT had been my home away from home for as long as I could remember. For sixteen years, Dad had dropped me off at Phillip's office every Thursday afternoon, and Mom picked me up half an hour later. The stretching session improved my mobility, even if only for the few hours that remained in the day … short-lived, but worth it.

Besides the times I was recovering from needle or surgical procedures, my therapy appointments were pretty predictable. Today, Patty, my newest PT, would stretch my legs like Phillip had—for roughly the first ten minutes of the session. I could easily notice an increase in flexibility before even taking a step away from the table. Phillip was famous for squirting a cool gel onto my kneecaps, and then with a little suction cup which looked like a mini plunger, he'd rapidly raise and lower my kneecap. I always enjoyed telling Mom that "Phillip suctioned my knees again," because she thought this sounded so painful. For the most part, it felt good. On rare occasions, a piece of cartilage would sneak into the suctioned area, which triggered a moment of pain. I'd wince a little, but it never hurt enough for me to say, "Hey, don't do that." On days when my spasticity had me all but in a ball, Phillip would place my arm at a forty-five-degree angle, then bounce it gently on the table. Within minutes, my tense muscles would be relaxed, and I would feel free again.

Today, as I think back to all the years of PT—all of the chauffeuring that my mother and father did to get me there—I can't believe it is over. Yes, Patty told me today, "You have graduated."

When I first met Patty two years ago, I couldn't walk into the rehabilitation center by myself. I held onto my mother's arm; every ounce of energy was needed to keep me from falling. After the typical new-patient paperwork, Patty had to conduct all of the therapy in a closed-door room. I feared people watching me, and the possibility of others bumping into me. I was at my weakest state, and I demanded privacy. Like Phillip, Patty would also have me lie down on a table to perform exercises like leg-lifts. But with Patty, no matter how hard I tried, I couldn't do them. She was so understanding and patient. She wanted to see me succeed and regain some independence, so she suggested that I use a cane or arm braces to help me walk. I feared these devices—they would be much too cumbersome and I'd eventually stumble and smack the floor. The amount of energy my body used to simply *get to* therapy far exceeded what I was getting out of it. So ... I quit.

Six months later, I walked back into Patty's office, alone and standing taller than ever before. The receptionist's face looked stunned. If I didn't know better, I would have thought she saw a ghost.

"What happened? You look fantastic!" she said in shock.

"I got a new diagnosis," I replied, beaming as if I went to the Mall of America to buy it.

I continued explaining that I lived the first thirty-three years of my life with the wrong diagnosis, "and now I can do so many things that I never could do before. I have been given an unbelievable gift," I added as I watched her jaw drop to the desktop.

Within a few sessions, Patty worked on things that I never imagined possible. At first, she had me revisiting the hip and leg raises, and all of the other exercises that I had grown up doing. She requested that I work out in the gym area of the rehabilitation center where I sat on a big blue exercise ball. That, in itself, made me smirk since, until recently, I could barely sit in a chair, even if it had arm supports.

Then she had my body continue balancing on the ball, belly up, while my legs crept forward. Finally, with my legs extended, and my knees bent to about a forty-five-degree angle, my neck remained resting on the ball. I stayed as flat as a table. It was a very difficult task the first few times, but I was doing it! Every muscle in my body felt engaged, and I loved it! *Thank you, God! I'm not sure if I deserve this. How can it be that I have muscles—I'm telling them what to do, and they're listening!* As our sessions continued, she pushed the envelope a little bit further. She had me get into the table position, and then she pushed on either side of my hips to offset my balance. Amazingly, I held my own.

We also worked on numerous other balancing exercises. She would time me as I stood on one leg, or as I balanced myself on a small teeter-totter device—two things that I couldn't have done in my wildest dreams a few months ago. Minutes flew by like seconds, and if I could have had my way, I would have camped out there for days, just to see what else could be mastered.

I called my mom as soon as I got home from my final session with Patty.

"Mom, I graduated from physical therapy!" I squealed. Mom's never been one to show her sensitive side, so I was surprised to hear tears in her voice.

"Did you ever think this day would come?" she asked.

I answered with my heart, "No, Mom."

Then I had to ask, "Did you?"

The Famous Doctor Will See You Now

When I was three, my mom was tired of watching me struggle with walking—although this didn't seem to stop me from having fun. When I attempted to keep up with my older brothers in the yard, I giggled and yelled their names as my curly pigtails flapped in the wind. Every time I fell to the grass, I got right back up and continued to chase the two older boys.

After seeing nearly a dozen doctors, my parents, Ann and Roger, knew that something wasn't right, so they scheduled an appointment for me to see Dr. Richard Anderson. He was arguably the best pediatric neurologist in the country. Unfortunately, we couldn't get in to see him for nearly six months.

Finally, as my parents waited in the pediatric neurology reception area, they noticed all the children in wheelchairs, and all the children with noticeable mental challenges. My dad looked at me as I sat on my mom's lap, with my pigtails and my bright smile as she read me a children's book. He thought how lucky he was that I was normal, with the exception of my scissor-walking. I could talk and laugh and was a very smart little girl, he thought. The wait for Dr. Anderson was just long enough for my father to quietly count his blessings.

Escorted to the examination room, we waited another hour and a half before the doctor who had written the books on pediatric neurology joined us. This was a draining day for both my parents.

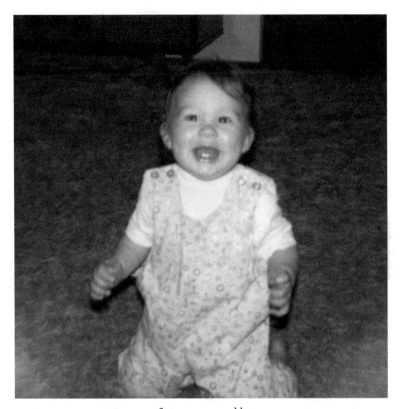

Jean, one year old

My mom entertained me by reading my favorite books, then saying "yes" when I asked to play with the chalkboard that hung on the wall. I finished a drawing of my family just as Dr. Anderson and a resident entered the room. The doctor wasted no time at all. He listened to my parents' concerns before thoroughly examining me. "Hop up on the table," he stated.

Dr. Anderson was an expressionless man. When I got older, I would ask my mom, "Why do I have to see him?" By then, I had been on the same medication for years, and truly hated these clinic visits. He would just stare at me and rub his chin. There wasn't anything friendly about him. My mom had the same reply every time, "We're not taking you there to make friends. He's the best, and he'll know

14

of any new medical developments before any other doctor." She was right … except for the whole misdiagnosis.

I struggled to hop on the table, but I was determined to do it on my own. When I reached the top of the examination table, I smiled proudly, revealing the dimples in my cheeks. As my mom looked at me, she understood why all of the nurses oohed and aahed over how cute I was. My olive skin, dark brown eyes, and curly pigtails were just a small part of my bubbly personality. My positive attitude and determination were so obvious; I made even complete strangers smile in my presence.

Dr. Anderson instructed me to "relax" as he gently shook my limbs, one by one. He checked my eyes with a small flashlight. Then he examined the dexterity of my fingers by having me pretend to play the piano. As asked, I brought my index finger to my nose, and then to his finger several times, alternating hands when told to do so. He reached for the reflex hammer and gently tapped the back of my heel cord with no results. Taking the sharp end of the medical device, he scraped the arc of my foot. I jolted as I grabbed for the side of the examination table—a result of the piercing pain through my foot.

"Let's see you walk," Dr. Anderson said to me.

I slowly climbed off of the table, and Dr. Anderson led me to the hallway. "Walk to the end of the hall and back." I did exactly as I was told and couldn't help but notice Dr. Anderson's black bushy eyebrows frowning as he inspected my gait.

"I need to get a better look at her legs while she walks. I'll need her to do this one more time, but this time in her underwear." He said, looking at my mom.

My mom took me back into the examination room and helped me take my pants off to reveal my favorite Strawberry Shortcake underwear. "You're doing a great job, Jeanie," my mom said with encouragement.

I took to the empty hallway one more time. Dr. Anderson now had a better view of the knees that knocked one another, and the tiptoes that forced me forward on a daily basis. He took notice of my left arm that bent up tightly to my side. He began to rub his chin as he watched me turn around to walk back toward the gawking group. We all walked back into the room. "I'd like to run a couple tests," Dr. Anderson stated bluntly. He muttered something to his resident, then shook my parents' hands as he left the room.

My parents and I headed to a different floor of the building. The male nurse asked my mom to put me in the white and blue robe for a CAT scan test. The nurse led us into a stale medical room with a long, narrow table. My dad set me on the table and kissed my forehead. "You're going to need to lie perfectly still, Jeanie. When we're done, we'll go out for lunch." He patted my leg and slowly exited the room with my mom, leaving me alone on the hard table.

The tech also explained to me that I needed to lie very still. He gently tightened a two-inch-wide strap around my forehead to ensure that I didn't move. He checked to make sure I was comfortable and then informed me that he would be on the other side of the window, "just for a few seconds."

I responded with a timid smile. Moments later, I felt the table moving me up into a big tube. Feeling like I just entered a cave, I turned my head to try to see what was going on. From the intercom, I heard the man's voice, "Stay still." I did as I was told, and was relieved when, a few minutes later, the table glided out of the tube again.

My parents took me to Perkins for lunch as promised. I ordered the Fancy Pants—a kid's meal consisting of pancakes covered in strawberries and whipped cream. I was beaming as I ate the treat, unaware that a tradition had just begun.

* * *

My parents continued to raise their family as they waited for the results of the CAT scan, only to find out that more tests were ordered. The unknown was killing my mom. She needed to know what was wrong with her little girl. *Please, God, give us answers. I can handle knowing what's wrong with my little girl, but I don't know how to deal with the unknown. How can it be that the best doctor can look at her and not have an answer?*

We found ourselves back at Dr. Anderson's for yet another test. Again, I was asked to lie on a sterile table, but this time my parents stayed by my side. My father stood up by my head and my mother stayed toward my feet. Looking at their brave little girl, a tech explained the test to all of us.

"They will be placing needles into the nerves of Jean's foot which will send electric currents through her legs. If she feels pain, it means her nerve endings work."

Without warning, the tech began with my right foot, which caused me to flinch with pain. "It hurts," I cried. The currents immediately went through my right foot again.

"This time I need you to tip your toes towards your head, sweetie," the tech informed me.

I obeyed the tech's request, and cried out in more pain. The cry was bittersweet to my daddy's ears.

"Okay," the tech said, "We're done with that foot. Now, we just have to do this on your left foot. Then we'll be all done."

"No," I whimpered as a tear rolled down my right cheek.

My dad bent down and whispered in my ear, "You squeeze my hand as much as you think it hurts, and then I'll feel the same amount of pain as you. If you do this today, I promise that you will never have to do this test again." He gently removed the tear from my cheek with his thumb.

"Okay," I looked at my dad with all the trust in the world.

The technician began again. I held my breath while squeezing my dad's rough hands as hard as I possibly could. My dad looked down at me, wishing it were he lying on the table, enduring this agony. *No amount of Perkin's Fancy Pants pancakes will make this memory go away.*

My parents and I endured a similar appointment with Dr. Anderson, so he could do another examination and observe me walk. He informed us that he would review the tests further, and would contact my parents as soon as he had a conclusive diagnosis.

The days of waiting turned into weeks. My mother continued to be the busy mom—my two brothers and I unaware of the turmoil she had building inside her. The unknown was far worse than hearing bad news. All the different scenarios played out in her head, like evil tricks, or nightmares. Yet, she carried on with life's chores as though nothing was wrong. Laundry was washed, dinners were made, the boys were delivered to their many activities … and I was treated as if nothing was wrong.

Then one day, the phone rang as my mom folded a load of bath towels on her double bed. She ran to answer it in the kitchen, and heard one of Dr. Anderson's residents on the other end.

"Hello, Mrs. Sharon?"

"Yes," she replied with a slight desperation in her voice.

The resident informed her that he was "calling on behalf of Dr. Anderson. I've been asked to inform you that we don't know what is wrong with your daughter. We don't have a conclusive diagnosis, and you should be prepared for anything—in fact, we can't be sure how long she will live."

The rest of the phone call didn't matter. All my mother heard was that the best doctor in the country didn't know what was wrong with me. *Not knowing what will happen—this is impossible. No one can live like this.* She quietly hung up the phone and walked back to her laundry. The pain was so deep, no amount of tears could possibly make her feel better.

By the time I was six years old, Dr. Anderson informed my parents that I had spastic diplegia. "I wanted to wait until I was certain that this diagnosis was correct." He explained that spastic diplegia meant two things: "Spastic represents the spasticity in the muscles and diplegia means that it affects both the arms and legs—yet one is worse than the other. In your daughter's case, her legs are worse." Dr. Anderson stressed that this was not a disorder that would get progressively worse. My parents found solace in knowing that as long as Dr. Anderson, the leader in pediatric neurology, oversaw my medical needs, they could cope with this news.

* * *

It was a bright and sunny Saturday morning. I had finished my morning chores of cleaning my bedroom, dusting the house, and unloading the dishwasher. I was free to do whatever I wanted. I didn't have plans to play with a friend, so I began snooping in the upstairs linen closet. This was just outside the family bathroom, located a few steps from my parents' bedroom, where my mom was putting clean sheets on her bed.

I opened the bifold door and saw the shelf for the sheets that would cover our four beds—three twin and one double, all located in the upstairs of our modified split-level home. My eyes glanced at my two older brothers' sheets that were brown and tan striped. My lips curved up in a slight smile as I remembered Christmas Eve from two years back.

We had returned home from five o'clock Christmas Eve mass to eat our family meal on the special holiday dishes that Tom and I had given Mom a year or two earlier. Mike, Tom, and I ran down the four steps to our burgundy-carpeted family room that hosted the biggest, greenest, and most decorated Christmas tree on Martin Court. Nearly two dozen gifts, beautifully wrapped in snowman and Santa Claus paper, were tucked under the tree. All three of us began searching for our names on each and every package. Moments later, Mom and Dad joined us in the family room.

"Mom, can we please open a present tonight?" Tom asked.

"No, you need to wait until the morning," she answered him with a smile.

"Please, Mom?" Mike pleaded.

"Please, just one." I joined in.

After our best begging, my dad spoke up.

"All right," he said. "We will let you each open a single gift on one condition. After you open your gift, you are not to say one word about it. I don't want to hear that you don't like it. If you do, we will never let you open a present on Christmas Eve again."

"Okay!" we quickly agreed.

"Jean, you can open yours first," my mom said, handing me my gift.

I tore into the package that was about the size of a Bible, but much lighter in weight ... Holly Hobbie makeup and perfume.

"Thank you so much!" I said, ripping into the box to get a closer look.

"My turn!" Mike and Tom said in unison.

"You can both open your gifts at the same time," my father said, handing them identical packages that appeared to be rather heavy.

"Okay!" they responded eagerly.

They both ripped open their packages with every ounce of energy they had. Their faces fell ... not a hint of gratitude could be seen.

"They got sheets!" I chuckled.

At that moment, they both grabbed their new sets of twin sheets, said "thank you," and strolled up to bed.

I shook my head and smiled as the memory came back in a flash, then I looked down to see all the Fisher Price Little People toys scattered on the floor of the closet. From the floor, my eyes gradually scanned clear up to the top shelf. *Easter baskets? Why would those be up there? Did the Easter bunny come back after we ate our candy and put them there for easy access?* I stood and thought about that for a moment, and knew in my heart what the answer was.

Just as I was about to close the closet door, I saw it. On the second shelf from the top, precisely the third item down on a stack of Mom's books was my baby book. I glanced toward my mom putting the sheets on her bed—still unaware of my snooping. I returned to the closet and stepped onto the bottom shelf, trying to reach the perfect height to grasp the book. I stretched as far as I could with my right hand, until the green book was in my grasp. *I've got it!*

I took the book around the corner to my own bedroom, and jumped on my yellow Holly Hobbie canopy bed. I opened the book and saw my name: Jean Ann Sharon, born on July 20, 1976. *This is it!* I saw my baby bracelet on one page, and my birth certificate on the other. Mom had filled in the first few pages with things that I never knew. For instance, I got my first tooth when I was seven months old, and a clump of my curly hair must have been cut about the same time. I turned the page and saw more of my mother's handwriting.

Jean's legs turn in as she walks, but the doctors tell me that this is something she will outgrow.

I took the book and ran into my mother's bedroom. My fear of being reprimanded for snooping had vanished.

"Mommy, this says that I'm going to outgrow my trouble walking! I'm not always going to walk like this," I said grinning from ear to ear as I went to sit on her freshly made bed.

Setting a bottle of perfume back on her dresser, Mom clenched the dust rag in her hand as she sat down beside me.

"I'm sorry, honey," she said as she turned towards me and took the book from my hands. "The doctor we saw when you were a toddler thought that you would outgrow the spasticity in your arms and legs, but that isn't right. You will have this forever, but you can keep praying when you go to church and maybe God will make you better."

"Okay," I said quietly. Leaving the baby book in her hands, I got up and slowly left Mom's room. I made my way back to my bedroom to play with my baby dolls and every Sunday I prayed for legs that would allow me to walk, run, and maybe someday play on a softball team.

As the mother of two lovable daughters, I don't like disappointing them with any change in plans, even if it is as simple as canceling a night at the movies, or calling off playtime in the park. I can't imagine how painful it was for my mother to look into my innocent eyes and shatter my sudden hopes—however brief they may have been.

At the time, I don't think it really occurred to me what I was missing in life. I hadn't a clue what it was like to run freely with friends on the playground. I hadn't learned to dribble a basketball down the court or slide into home plate. It didn't matter to me what strangers thought as they stared while I walked down the toy isle in Kmart.

What mattered was that my mom was there for me when I needed her most. She would drop everything to cheer me up when I came home to say that someone had imitated my walking that day. She would often say that "everyone gets made fun of for something," and the only thing that they had on me was that I had a different walk. She'd remind me how friendly and beautiful I was.

"They're just jealous, Jean," she'd reassure me.

I know that our relationship would have been different had I been "normal." I joke with her now, and tell her, "Without my funny walk, I would have been a brat." I was pretty and fun to be around, so I would have hung out with the popular kids at school—those who were tortured by peer pressure. I can't help but think of my physical abnormality as a gift from God. Yes, being a spastic ball allowed me to be close to my parents not only because I needed them, but because they were fun! I have no regrets that they were two of my closest friends.

Yet, my parents did everything they could to make me a strong, bubbly, optimistic, and *normal* girl. They never said that I couldn't do activities, and they pushed me to try new things. I was a Girl Scout, I took ceramics classes, and my mom always urged me to call friends to play for the afternoon.

When I was fourteen, I went to school sporting events with my parents every Friday night. They would make me walk what seemed like a mile to get to the metal bleachers. While their adult friends said they were being mean to me—they should wheel me to my seat—my mom would inform them that I could make it. My parents knew it would take me triple the time, but they wanted me to strengthen my muscles. Had they given up on me and put me in a wheelchair full-time, I don't know that I would have ever gotten all my strength back after my new diagnosis.

While growing up, there were times that I would ask God, *Why me? Why doesn't Tom have any difficulty walking? Why do I have it so much worse than Mike?* It never seemed fair that Mike ultimately had my same diagnosis, took the same amount of medication as me, yet his impairment went unnoticed by others. Sure, he wasn't able to play as many sports as he wanted to, but he could go to the store and not feel the eyes of strangers on him. He could participate in phys ed at school without looking like the least athletic kid on the court.

For whatever reason, I was born with spasticity. There wasn't anything I could do about it. I had to work hard to do the little things in life that others took for granted. I never understood how my friends were capable of running, walking, skipping, or just going from point A to point B without giving it a thought. It didn't take me long to realize that life was good no matter what angle I saw it from. Rather than put my energy into what I couldn't do, I learned to fight, work hard, and conquer what was possible. No one's growing-up years are easy … mine just seemed like something *no one* was prepared to handle.

Camping Out
for a Second Opinion

REFUGE FROM ALL OF THE CLINIC CONCERNS CAME FROM the most basic family events. For instance, simple things like family dinners and Friday night movies, vacations and short weekend trips—these things still trigger my strongest appreciation for family when I think back to my preteen years. Time with Mom, Dad, and my brothers brought simple sanctuary from medical schedules.

Any break from doctors was welcomed, since by the time I was six years old I wasn't only seeing Dr. Anderson every six months. My regular clinic visits were trumped up by Dr. O'Neil, a physiatrist who focused on how to minimize my tiptoe and knock-knee walking. Dr. O'Neil, a sweet and patient man, was a nerve, muscle, and bone expert who taught me many new stretches. Some I could do at home—either on my own or with my mom or a brother's help.

Each day started off with the heel-cord stretch. The dark, knee-high mark on the living room wall—my shoe hitting just the right spot—was proof that a day didn't go by without this five-minute maneuver performed on each leg. When I asked Dr. O'Neil, "How long will I have to do this exercise?" he smiled and said, "Until you're seventeen." He knew … he must have … that by the time I reached my teens, I'd *want* to do this stretch as often as possible, so daily life would be just a little easier.

One cold winter morning, my mom took me from my first-grade class for a special visit to Dr. O'Neil. His plan: To put both my feet in casts. This would stop my spastic tiptoe stance, which would in turn improve my walking.

In our bulky winter coats, Mom and I walked down the long hospital hallway. I always slowed my pace when we reached the massive mural of smiling kids. The dozen or so children in the painting all looked so different from my classmates at Crooked Lake Elementary. They were black, white, Asian, and Hispanic. My favorite child in the picture was the little blonde girl on the end. With curly pigtails, she shared a bright smile even though she was in a wheelchair. She reminded me of … me, at a time when I really didn't think there were any kids in the world like me. It makes me sad now—imagining one of my daughters having these thoughts … of any child being alone in her *condition*. But at the time, I just considered this my private appraisal of the mural—one that I would guard in my mind, and keep to myself. Perhaps my mom read my mind as I slowed down to the pace of a turtle every time we meandered past this familiar display. But she never asked. So, I scanned the mural for the little girl, as if to see how she was doing, then continued toward Dr. O'Neil's office.

As we stepped past her that day, I thought about how lucky I was. No matter how difficult for me, I still *walked* the long hallway. *That girl can't. I bet she'll never chase her brothers around the house or go sledding down the hill. She probably can't ever ride a bike. I still need my training wheels, but at least I can ride a bike.*

Dr. O'Neil entered the room where Mom and I had been waiting for a while. "Sit on the table, Jean." My quickness had improved, so I no longer needed to use the step at the end of the table. I climbed up in my most agile way, excited for the procedure. As he ran through the familiar checks—tests that Dr. Anderson typically did—Dr. O'Neil smiled and occasionally asked, "How are you doing?" I recall thinking, *He seems happy to see me. I think he cares about me and Mom.*

Dr. O'Neil prepared us, "Okay, I'm going to put casts on both of your feet." He showed me the rolling tray next to the table where he had everything he would need: the rolled plaster, a bowl of water, scissors, and socks that I was asked to put on first.

"Are you ready?" Dr. O'Neil inquired with a smile.

I nodded; my eyes gave away my excitement. *I'm about to get casts!*

Dr. O'Neil gently pulled the thin white socks over each of my feet. He picked up a long piece of casting material, dipped it in the bowl of water, then slowly wrapped the wet fabric around my right foot. He continued to do this until one foot was covered from calf to toes, of course leaving a window for my little piggies to wiggle and breathe. He repeated the procedure, and quickly covered my left calf and foot as well. He tapped my bare knee, letting me know that I did a good job.

Dr. O'Neil turned to my mom and stated, "Now, she can't walk on these for another hour or so. They need to completely dry. Call if you have any concerns, or notice any difficulties with the casts."

My mom nodded in agreement and Dr. O'Neil suggested that she pull up the car. Moments later, the doctor scooped me up and placed me in the backseat. We were on our way home with my funny new footwear.

"Can we go out to lunch?" I asked, even though I already knew my mom's answer. We always ate lunch somewhere fun after an Anderson or O'Neil appointment.

Thirty minutes later Mom pulled the white Chevrolet into the Coon Rapids McDonald's.

"Don't get out of the car," my mom stated in a concerned tone. "You can't walk on those casts yet; I'll have to carry you."

My mom exited the car and opened the backseat passenger door. She grabbed me from my seat and cradled me in her arms like I was an infant. I wrapped my arms around her neck to help her support my weight. It all came so naturally, even though my mother hadn't carried me in years. I was just too heavy, now that I was seven. But suddenly she had Wonder Woman strength.

Just as she closed my car door, we heard an older woman's voice, "Oh, no ... both legs!" We saw a thin, white-haired old lady walking by us with a stunned look on her face.

I laughed in my mother's ear, "She thinks I broke both of my legs!"

While I ate my cheeseburger Happy Meal, I heard the repeated alarm of the little old lady's voice in my head. If she only knew the real story. Two broken legs would be welcomed by comparison to the real reason for my casts. My mom looked at me and asked, "What's so funny?"

"She thinks I broke both of my legs. I can't wait to tell Daddy that one," I said, taking the last bite of my burger.

After a few short weeks of the casts, my parents and I knew this treatment would not be a success. The plan was for the casts to keep me off of my toes … to force me to use my heels more. Yet, because of the casts, I wasn't able to walk at all!

At school, I sat on my teacher's desk chair so the kids could wheel me where I needed to go. And at home, I crawled around the house like a toddler, reluctant to walk.

Dr. O'Neil agreed with my parents—this was not his objective.

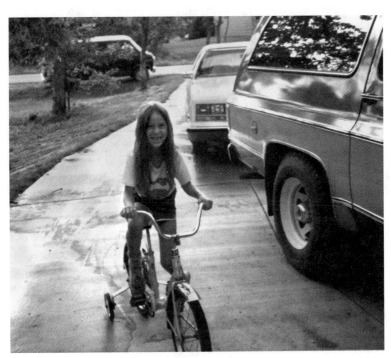

Jean learning to ride a bike

My mom took me back to his office and he sawed off both casts. He wasn't about to give up on me, however. Dr. O'Neil handed my mom my casts, along with some ace bandages.

"I want you to put these on her every night before bed."

He explained that this would help stretch my heel cord at night and hopefully I could walk less on my toes, engaging my heels. At the time, I believed I would end up doing this for a month or two. To my surprise, these casts became my new nighttime accessories—*forever.* I was wrapped like a mummy from knees to toes every night, until one year—probably because I had grown so much—my dad had me fitted for plastic casts. These orthoses, secured by Velcro straps, created more independence for me. By the time I entered my teen years, I could put them on by myself at bedtime.

Not long after I had my casts cut off, I decided to conquer my bike. Every kid wants to learn how to ride, and I was no different. All of my friends could ride their bikes *without* training wheels, and I desperately wanted to be like them. Tom had been helping me off and on, for two years! One would think, by the age of seven, I could ride a two-wheeler.

I must say, Tom tried everything.

"Come on, Jean. Don't be afraid. It'll work." I tried to keep my balance in the yard where there was no pavement to fear. "If you fall," Tom said, "the grass will cushion the blow when you hit the ground." Of course, I hit—faster than either of us imagined.

"Okay. Let's try this," Tom persevered. "Ride down the hill through the grass." I must have looked a little frightened, because Tom urged me on. "It's just our yard—it's not the Rocky Mountains." He cheered as I steered down the backyard incline, thinking the speed would keep my momentum going. But I failed at this technique too. I fell to the ground, scraping my arms and knees. "I think I need some Band-Aids," I observed.

Tom didn't give up. And I cooperated with every new idea he formulated.

His current theory would take some time to test. "Jean, you can do this," Tom said, giving me yet another round of encouragement.

Tom raised my training wheels a little bit every week. Over the next few weeks of the summer, Tom had me ride my bike as often as possible. I was clearly getting stronger. My speed and balance were improving!

I rode my bike faithfully, every morning. Luckily, we lived on a cul-de-sac with only three houses. I kept riding around and around the dead-end street. I got faster and faster, riding for longer periods of time each day that I practiced. I didn't let the hot July sun get to me.

One late afternoon, our neighbor stopped by to talk with Dad. As she explained it, "I can see her out my living room window. Her training wheels don't ever touch the ground. I'm sure they can come off now." She stated this so matter-of-factly that Dad wondered if Helen was in charge of this plot to make me a bike rider.

Could it be? Is it possible that my days of riding a baby bike are over?

"Go—get on your bike." Dad took a good look as I rode it, balanced on the two wheels.

"Pull over, Jeanie." Tom and I stood close by as Dad grabbed a tool and wrenched the training wheels right off my bike.

"Okay. Try it again, Jeanie," Dad stated, still in his dirty drywall clothes.

I jumped on the mauve-colored banana seat. I'd loved this bike from the first moment I saw it in the driveway—a birthday gift two years ago.

"I'll give you a good push," Dad stated. "Pedal as fast as you can." I couldn't look at Tom—all of my focus had to go into this ride. But I knew my brother was watching and rooting for me.

"Here we go," Dad cheered as he gave me a firm push. I started down the concrete driveway, but felt an immediate change as his strong hand let go.

I pedaled just like Dad said—as fast as I could! *I am still upright!* At the end of the driveway, I steered to my left, doing my regular route around the cul-de-sac. *I am riding my bike!!!*

I kept pedaling and pedaling, a smile plastered to my face. I felt my hair blowing behind me. *This is so cool!* I made my way back into the driveway and realized that despite the two years of Tom's teaching, we never once discussed how to avoid falling over when the bike came to a stop. *I don't care. I can ride my bike! That's all that matters to me.* I steered my bike from the concrete to the lawn, and let myself crash, falling onto my left side.

I crawled from under the weight of the bike, and squealed with excitement. "I did it!"

I don't know if I have ever seen two faces look so proud. Thinking back, I wonder if Tom would have coached me in bike-riding 101 for another seven years. I have a strange feeling he would have, as long as I continued to try. But at this point, we all took a grateful step back in quiet celebration of what just happened.

"Let's go show Alex and Matt!" Tom said, referring to the neighborhood boys who lived a couple of streets away.

Tom grabbed his bike, and the two of us rode off down the street—together. We pulled up to Alex and Matt's split-level home where they were playing in their driveway. That's when I realized for the second time that day, I hadn't been taught how to stop. I turned awkwardly onto their grass and fell, a little more gracefully this time.

Alex came running up to me, a big smile on his face, looking almost as proud as Tom. A really good friend since kindergarten, Alex included me when he played boy games like cops and robbers. His mom was so nice—we knew the whole family would be happy for me.

"Your training wheels are gone!" he announced, looking at my bike.

Tom and I described our day and all of the details leading up to my first true bike ride. Tom did most of the talking since I was too excited to explain. *I learned how to ride my two-wheeler, so that's exactly what I want to do.* Alex and Matt joined us. We rode back to our house and rounded the cul-de-sac a few more times.

Quarter to five couldn't come soon enough. That's when I could share my new talent with the one other person who would exult in this moment. I waited outside until my mom's white Chevy pulled into the driveway. Tom stood right beside me because this was just as big a deal to him as it was to me.

"Mom, we've got something to show you!" we yelled to her before she could even get out of the car. Looking tired from the long day at work, she crawled out of the driver's seat wearing her work clothes—dress pants and a blouse. She couldn't ignore our excitement, so instead of going straight into the house, she patiently waited for us.

I ran from the garage—I moved toward my bike as fast as my body would let me, on tiptoes, legs slightly turned in. I wasn't about to let my slow approach to the bike stop me from showing off for Mom.

For what must have been the fiftieth time that day, I hopped on my bike and rode down the driveway, imagining the awe in my mother's face. I rode as fast as I could down the street, around the cul-de-sac, and back. When I returned and dropped my bike in the yard—a planned fall this time—I looked up to see Mom waiting, watching, smiling—tears in her eyes and giving thanks to the heavens. *If I didn't know better, this might be the happiest day of her life.*

* * *

My bike riding skills, though exciting, did not erase the fact that at Crooked Lake Elementary School I was a "special education" student—at least from a physical fitness standpoint. Two special-ed teachers pulled me regularly from my classmates. Mr. Jones, who let me call him Chris, seemed cool, and picked activities I enjoyed. But I didn't love my time with him. *He treats me like a baby*, was my thought when he asked me to perform skills that any kindergartner could do. Yet, there were times when he let me do things that only older students or adults could do—then praised me for doing it better.

One week, he took me outside to play football. *Football?!* I thought. But then I considered—*that's the unit the rest of my class is doing in regular phys ed.* I was suddenly pumped for this plan to go outside and show off my quarterbacking skills. I loved throwing a football. *I think I'm the best girl at throwing a spiral ... in my class, anyway.*

I put on my fall jacket, and Mr. Jones and I went out to the playground. I was a little worried about the temperature. *The crisp air isn't too cold. My muscles shouldn't tighten up too much.* Then, Mr. Jones

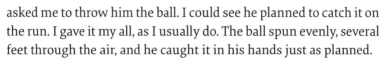

asked me to throw him the ball. I could see he planned to catch it on the run. I gave it my all, as I usually do. The ball spun evenly, several feet through the air, and he caught it in his hands just as planned.

"Wow," he smiled. "I don't think I could ever throw like that."

Hmmm … I may not be able to walk well, but my brain works fine. I'm fully aware that you are able to throw a football better than that. You're a phys ed teacher. Mr. Jones—Chris—was a really nice guy, but I didn't like being patronized. I lacked the assertiveness to share my sarcastic thoughts … but I wished I could have explained. *At home I am pushed—I'm expected to keep up with every able-bodied person. No one would be impressed by that spiral. The Vikings' quarterback has nothing to worry about.*

My favorite physical activities were practiced with Jennifer, my school's physical therapist. It seemed natural to call her by her first name. Jennifer was equal parts friendly, happy, and pretty. Plus, she never gave me any breaks. I felt excitement whenever I spotted her standing at my classroom door. She stretched my muscles, like Phillip from PT. Yet, when she worked on my legs, she talked to me, and encouraged me to share everything about my day. I never saw her without a smile on her face, which brightened my outlook completely.

One day, as Jennifer and I walked to the cafeteria, where we held our impromptu phys ed sessions, she told me she was going to teach me to roller-skate. I looked at her wide-eyed, and her own blue eyes smiled back at me. *So, walking is difficult for me, and you're going to put wheels under my feet!* She must have read my mind because she began to explain, "It'll take a while, but I have a plan."

When we arrived in the cafeteria, I spotted a chair with roller skates parked on the seat. I looked at her with an anxious smile on my face, waiting for her instruction. Jennifer informed me that I would hold onto the chair while pushing myself forward slowly.

"It's going to take time, but you'll catch on." *If anyone else asked me to do this, I doubt if I'd even try. But if Jennifer thinks I can …* "Are these skates for me?"

Jennifer eagerly helped me out of my shoes, slid my feet into each brown skate, and had me tie them securely. As she pulled me up to my feet, she positioned the chair so that I could balance myself as I stood upright. The chair seemed perfect for my height. "Hang on to the back of it," Jennifer reminded me.

At first, I practiced standing so I could get used to the wheels under my feet. Jennifer was right within reach of me, just in case I fell. "I'm not worried about falling," I stated confidently. Suddenly, I wanted to skate!

Jennifer coached me, "If you slowly slide the chair forward, then scoot your feet to catch up to the chair, you'll be skating!" I followed her directions to a T. Not only was I standing, but I was moving on wheels!

Jennifer and I worked on this task for over a month. Progress was slow, but I was improving. One day, as we entered the cafeteria, Jennifer announced, "You've been doing great. You're ready to try it without the chair."

Fear crossed my mind, but Jennifer was right there. I knew she only wanted the best for me. I smiled eagerly and gave her all of my trust. After I pulled myself up on my wheels, Jennifer pulled the chair that had been my support for so many weeks. I stood independently, frozen in time and space, panning the open cafeteria.

I didn't budge. This was good news, I guess, because it meant I hadn't fallen—yet. I slowly made my move. I slid my right foot forward. Again, to my surprise, I remained upright. My vision of Bambi, falling to his icy splits, twirling around on the frozen pond, began to fade. I let my left foot catch up with my right, moving forward ever so slightly. I repeated these steps until I was robotically, yet without a doubt, skating a slow circle around the cafeteria.

"You've got it!!" Jennifer cheered.

I was afraid to stop—to even think about what I was doing—so I didn't. I just kept repeating the motion, as I focused on not falling.

"Let's roller-skate back to your room so you can show your classmates," Jennifer said enthusiastically.

I followed Jennifer out of the cafeteria, and skated down the hallway toward my classroom. I was beaming. *I bet I'm the first kid to roller-skate in the halls. Nothing is going to get me down today!* I entered my fifth-grade classroom with skates on my feet, and slowly rode to my desk. All the kids stood up with big smiles on their faces, and I could tell they were just as happy for me as I was for myself.

"You're roller-skating, Jean!" Traci Bollinger said with a huge smile.

I took that moment to roller-skate around the room, not once, but twice, as Traci and others cheered me on.

* * *

In my final year at Crooked Lake Elementary School, I decided to play the clarinet in band. We practiced once a week in the cafeteria and I enjoyed it, even though I felt I wasn't very good. We had a band concert planned, and we each would be playing a duet. Mr. Taylor announced our duet partners—my classmate Amy and I would be playing our song together. We practiced our song in and outside of school—we knew we were prepared.

Once the concert date was officially set, Amy explained to me, "I have a softball game that night. I can't perform at the concert. Sorry." *How am I going to play a duet without her? Maybe I won't have to play my song. Maybe Mr. Taylor won't have me play at all.* But once Mr. Taylor learned that Amy could not be there for the concert, he turned to me and said, "You can play your song as a solo." Tears came to my eyes, but I couldn't let them fall. *Mr. Taylor can't make me do this alone. I'll just pray. God, you've given me enough to deal with in life. Isn't it bad enough that I can't keep up with kids on the playground? Please, just this once, give me the easy way out! Don't make me go through this solo. Please, God. Help Mr. Taylor to understand that I can't do this alone! He has to change his mind the night of the concert.*

Two weeks later, I was at school, ready for the band concert. We prepared three songs together as a group, then our duets would be showcased—except for me, I hoped.

Suddenly, my muscles tensed up, and my stomach began to flip-flop. I wasn't sure, but I thought I was going to be sick. Moments later, we all walked out together and took our places at the front of the gym. As I scanned the audience, our parents looked anxious to hear how far we had come in band.

After our group songs, Mr. Taylor introduced each duet. Of course, when it was my turn, he explained to the crowd that "Jean was supposed to play a duet tonight, but her partner was unable to attend. Jean will be playing her duet as a solo." He seemed to go on and on about how my duet was now a solo, making me more and more nervous by the minute! *Come on, God! I thought you'd give me a break this one time! I should be grateful ... he's bracing everyone for a horrible clarinet song.*

My body began to shake from nervousness. I held my clarinet tightly in my hands and looked at the music in front of me. *I can get through this ... I have to get through this.* I played my first note and it came out as a very loud *squeak.* I heard a girl laugh from the back of the gym, and my nervousness doubled! I continued to shake as my piece played on. Half of the notes came out as squeaks, and by the time I finished the short song, tears were running down my cheeks. *I have embarrassed myself—not only from playing absolutely horrible music, but by crying in front of a gym full of parents.* It was not all the parents I cared about though—it was *my* parents. I knew that I had let them down.

After the concert, my face was still hot with tears. I wasn't sure if I ever would be able to face my classmates again. *Maybe I can be homeschooled?* When I approached my parents afterward, I could see the anger in their faces. I knew they didn't care that I stunk at playing my piece ... but they *did* care that I cried. *I have let everyone down, including myself. How could I have let myself cry? I'm so much stronger than this. Lord, please help me accept what I cannot change.*

As I slowly walked out of the gym with my head down, I saw Jeremy, another classmate, running toward me. He wasn't attempting to cheer me up. He was simply a boy with a mission to leap from the ground and touch the low ceiling. Our eyes suddenly met, and we realized that we were about to collide. When his feet hit the ground he landed smack on top of me, knocking me flat on my back. Springing to his feet again, Jeremy put his hands on my shoulders, then asked, "Are you okay?" He was so concerned that he had hurt me. Little did I know that my mom witnessed all of this. She would forever tease me about Jeremy hugging me after the concert. *I'm not sure if this night could get any worse.*

* * *

I think I was about eight when my brother Mike began showing symptoms like mine. At least that's what my parents told Dr. Anderson. Mike began coming with me to my neurology appointments where we did all of the same tests for spastic diplegia. The rubber-hammer test checked for a quick response at all the traditional reflex points. The hand-jive test—our nickname for a task I absolutely hated—required that, with hands positioned in my lap, I flip my palms as fast as possible. Palms down, palms up, palms down, palms up ... my hands could not coordinate this action in a symmetrical way.

Of course, there were other tasks, and while I struggled with some, Mike seemed to complete each test flawlessly. *What's he doing here? I'd give up a Barbie to have even one appointment where I could show off like that! ...* Until he had to stand on one leg. Mike just could not do this. He lost his balance every time.

So, you failed one test—not a big deal. I wanted to say this, but I was afraid to—especially since I wasn't sure how Mike felt about being compared to *me.* We left the clinic that day with knowledge that Dr. Anderson confirmed: We *both* had spastic diplegia.

Over time, I could see that Mike was anything but annoyed by having the same condition as me. He was almost apologetic when he performed Dr. Anderson's tests with ease. In fact, he always went second with these clinical tasks—as if everyone knew, "There's no way she can follow that act." Mike's sympathetic smile when I botched the hand jive always helped me comply with the next request. We never talked about it, but I sensed that he felt lucky ... and perhaps, on those clinic days, a little sorry that his sister had it worse.

Together, Mike and I continued to go to the neurologist twice a year. Recently, I found out that my parents had to pay for many of these clinic appointments out of their own pockets because the insurance would not cover them. Mom and Dad said they could handle the high costs of the appointments, but it was the prescriptions that threatened to break the bank. At a dollar per pill, eleven pills per day—*times two*—two children with this diagnosis would empty the family wallet fast.

When the financial stress heightened, my mom finally shared this information with our family practitioner. He told Mom to bring Dr. Anderson's written prescriptions to him. He would rewrite them and we could submit the costs to our family insurance. This worked since he was a provider covered under our health insurance.

I don't know how my parents survived the stress of all these medical worries while facing the growing financial burden of not one, but two, children in and out of clinics. Growing up, I never knew a thing about the financial aspects of our medical needs. Was I a selfish kid, clueless to all the expenses that come with good care? Was I that self-absorbed?

And we weren't exactly millionaires. I should have known that Mom and Dad worked hard for everything our family valued—our home, vacations, good meals, special holidays, school supplies, warm winter clothing, sports fees for my brothers ... Was I so detached that I didn't consider the conversations my parents had behind closed doors, where hardship was analyzed, and problems were tackled?

Or, were my parents just really good at guarding their children from more hardship? Did they work that diligently at sheltering us from the worry that comes from having a medically fragile child? There were never fights about what treatments I should receive. As far as I can recall, the two of them were always on the same page. They clearly shared the same mantra: *Do whatever it takes to allow our children to have the best lives possible.*

Dr. Anderson may have been the best neurologist out there, but my parents didn't take any chances. They also took me to the hospital that was known throughout the Midwest, if not the country. It was just too close to home to ignore. Its world-renowned reputation for having the best and the brightest on staff lured my parents to request a second opinion.

Once again, this would not be covered by our insurance. So, Mom and Dad made some creative plans when they heard that Mike and I would have to be in and out of tests for a full week. We took a camping trip to southern Minnesota—a family vacation, interrupted by daily appointments and tests with a slew of doctors I had never met before. Test after test made for long days. I tuned out most of the conversations between my parents and the physicians. However, my ears perked up when I heard, "We'd like to run the nerve test." The nerve conduction velocity test, that is.

I'm sure it was telepathy. One look at Dad, and he read my eyes: *I can't do that again. You promised me. Remember? God, please help him to remember!*

"Jean's already had that test; we won't be doing that again," my father said firmly.

By the end of the week, the physicians concluded what Dr. Anderson had said all along. "Quite honestly, he taught us everything about pediatric neurology," one doctor shared. When the team of physicians consults the books for anything regarding spastic diplegia, they find research and data from none other than Dr. Anderson. "He's the authority … he tracks this condition more than anyone."

I resigned myself to the facts: *I have spastic diplegia. There is no doubting that. And it will always be worse than my brother's. I will continue to take eleven baclofen pills a day. I will be in physical therapy for the rest of my life. And, more than likely, I will have more hospital visits in my future. All of this is out of my control, so Lord, I please ask you to guide me in accepting everything that I can't control and strength to live through it in a positive light.*

It Takes a Family

Dr. O'Neil moved out east and Dr. Byrd took his place. He, too, was a friendly, caring doctor. Since Dr. O'Neil had us on a good routine of stretching my heel cords, Dr. Byrd focused his attention on my knees—some strange magnetic force still brought them together with every step. Dr. Byrd strongly advised that I have shots in each groin to stop the knock-knee spasticity. He called the shots "blocks" since the injections stopped my knees from crossing one another while in stride.

"The blocks sound like a good idea, Jeanie," my dad explained.

So, at the age of seven, I was put under anesthesia for the very first time because of the precision needed for this outpatient treatment. I had the choice of being put to sleep by needle or gas, but what kid likes the prick of the needle? I opted for the gas.

Over the course of six years, I was knocked out for the blocks four times. The first two times, I asked for the gas mask, but found myself vomiting as soon as I woke up. The third time, I decided to be strong. I took the pinch in my arm like a pro. All four times, I walked out of the hospital without the fear of my knees even kissing one another. However, as I aged and my body grew, the blocks didn't seem to work as well. Walking improved with each application of the drug, but for shorter periods of time. It seemed futile to even try the process again, the relief was so short-lived.

After the fourth block, Dr. Byrd advised my parents to "consider a muscle transfer. Jeanie should see Dr. Christensen." This surgeon specialized in a process where the muscles from one part of each leg were detached, then reattached to a different part of each leg. "This will permanently stop her knees from hitting one another."

Dr. Byrd joined us for our consult with Dr. Christensen. Dr. Byrd wanted to make sure that the surgeon understood exactly what my needs were … and that my parents understood this horrific, yet helpful procedure. Dr. Byrd finished his explanation with, "And she'll be in a body cast for a month."

On the drive home from Dr. Christensen's, I sat quietly in the back seat of our car. The imagery of this surgery finally got the best of me, and I blurted out to my parents, "Can you believe that he thinks we'd actually do that?"

I watched my mom look at my dad. She held his silent gaze for a moment, then turned to face me in the seat directly behind Dad.

"You are going to have this surgery." Her solemn authority told me all the protest in the world would not change her mind.

A horror film played in my head as I visualized someone cutting my leg muscles off of my body. Sure, someone sewed them back on, like a rag doll who lost her legs to a mad dog. But I wanted the images to end. I knew I wouldn't win a battle against Mom, especially since Dad didn't raise one word of protest. He never even questioned my mother, who was adamant about the procedure. As I turned and looked out the window, I prayed that it would all be worth it.

* * *

That seventh-grade hiatus, when I shared the hospital room with crying babies, resulted in the body cast that Dr. Byrd had promised. Three days following surgery, my sleepless nights ended with an ambulance ride back home. As I looked out the window of the emergency vehicle while being backed into my driveway, I noticed the cellophane balloons tied to the mailbox. Bouncing in the breeze, one read, "Welcome Home," while the other had a picture of a white cat on it.

Grandma, Tom, and Tom's friend Kurt were in the driveway with smiles on their faces. They waved as the EMTs hauled me out of the ambulance and rolled the stretcher to the front door. It hadn't dawned on me at the time that almost a month would lapse before I'd see Mom's flower garden or smell the freshly cut lawn that Dad tried so desperately to keep green. When the front door shut behind us, I would be cooped up from the natural world until I returned to the hospital to have the cast cut off.

The EMTs parked me in the family room on a rented rolla-way bed. This similar setup to my upstairs bedroom included my nightstand—a cat-and-dog-papered photo box that held a bubble gum–colored clock radio and petite pink lamp. During my sleepless nights in the hospital, I spent plenty of time visualizing a month of solitary confinement in my room upstairs. I liked my room, but it seemed sad and lonely to be stuck there throughout my recovery. *I didn't think that I would be sleeping next to the big patio doors, right in front of the brick fireplace! This'll be good.*

Those recovery weeks went by so quickly. I was the center of attention. I received cards and gifts in the mail, and it seemed as though a new visitor arrived each and every day, usually with some sort of gift. Aunt Winnie came to visit, offering to help my mom. She gave me the coolest white T-shirt with a vibrant design of neon pink, green, and peach swirls, with matching socks. My cousin's wife, Sherry, came by with their new baby, Brent. *He's so cute.* Sherry even left him in his car seat next to my bed so I could watch him while she went into the kitchen to visit with Grandma.

Our house had a revolving front door. Every night I had a different friend come over to visit, even if it was just for an hour. My friends would give me the scoop on everything I was missing at school. Time flew with all of this activity.

Since the surgery took place in May, I missed a month of Fred Moore Junior High. This made the pain worthwhile! A tutor came to the house twice a week to give me all my assignments, and to help me with my questions. My guidance counselor made the decision that I would not need to take any of my finals since I'd "been through enough." My social studies teacher thought differently and demanded that I take the seventh-grade final for his class. I lay flat on my back in bed as I circled what I thought were the appropriate answers. Truthfully, I didn't care how I came out on the exam. Like my friends, I was eager to be done with school, especially since the last month was accomplished on a rollaway bed.

Once a week, my mom would announce that we should wash my hair. I would beg her to just leave it as it was. "It will be fine," I assured her. She would insist, and Grandma would help her place a sheet under me. When the bedding was ready, she would call for my dad and my brothers. Mike, a senior in high school, and Tom, a sophomore, would get on one side of the bed; my father would stand on the other. The three of them would grab hold of the sheet with both hands to lift me up.

"One, two, three, lift," Dad announced.

Hovering over the bed, I would begin my trek toward the kitchen, climbing ten careful steps to the sink. As they took the stairs, I prayed that they would not drop me. There was absolutely no extra space between them and the stairwell walls. I was at their mercy, suspended on the sheet between them, studying their confident faces while I held my breath. When the steps were completed, and the floor leveled out again, I could breathe. They walked me another ten steps, and slowly set me on the kitchen counter so that my head would reach the sink. They would slide me up so my mom could have my head under the faucet.

She used the sprayer to wash my bed-matted hair. She shampooed it, not once, but twice, and finished with just a drop of conditioner. As soon as she combed my hair, I anticipated the journey back down the stairs to my rollaway. The butterflies in my stomach would finally stop their fluttering. Thinking back, I don't know what seemed worse: climbing up or going down. But while Mom combed my hair, I used my usual line on Dad:

"Please, Daddy, just carry me down to bed," I would plead. *Dad's so strong; I know he can do it alone, without the boys—without any trouble.*

"Your cast is too heavy and you're dead weight in it, Jean." I'm sure my dad was afraid he might lose his balance on the steps and drop me.

"Please," I whimpered.

He called for my brothers and we performed the circus act once again. The boys never banged me against the stairwell walls in my makeshift hammock. But I envisioned this every time. By the third week of my captivity, Dad gave in … he carried me, cast and all, up and down the stairs.

We spent a lot of time in the family room that spring. I would lie in bed by the patio doors, but sometimes the bed was moved, rolled at an angle, so I could watch TV closer to everyone else. There was absolutely no movement on my part. As immobile as I stayed, day after day, my personal plumbing began to clog. I was given everything from prune juice to suppositories with no "success." I was a time bomb, ready to blow. It was not humanly possible to consume all this medical and organic *assistance* without some dramatic end.

On Monday night, we were finishing part two of the made-for-TV miniseries *I Know My First Name Is Steven*, when it hit me. "I have to poop," I told my mom. Tom and Mike disappeared. The room cleared fast. Then Mom, without looking away from the TV, asked me, "Can you just hold it for the last five minutes of the movie?" These were the days before the convenience of DVR.

"Now wait just a minute," Dad spouted, getting up from his chair. "You have been filling her to the brim with prune juice and laxatives. AND she's had suppositories. You cannot ask her to wait." With that, he left the room so my mom and Grandma could get me onto the bedpan.

* * *

My parents finally drove me to the hospital to have my cast removed. Tilted up on the examination table, with my mom sitting next to me, a doctor I had never met greeted me with his little saw in hand. I recognized this tool. I wondered to myself, *Does he ever get that thing sharpened?* As he began to cut the cast, this doctor must have read my mind. He suddenly announced, "We need to take the top half of the cast off … I'm going to let the nurse do this, and I will be back in just a few minutes."

When the door closed behind him, the nurse walked over and removed the top shell of my plaster pod. She and my mom helped me into my underwear and then we waited for the doctor to return. He said that he needed to check my skin to "be sure there aren't any sores. They can occur when pressure builds up between the cast and the skin." As he began looking, he warned, "Now, don't look down."

Of course, I looked—and when I spotted my left thigh, I saw an open purple wound about the size and shape of a Lay's Classic potato chip. That's when I looked away—I felt the faintness coming on fast, so I took his advice and rolled my eyes toward the ceiling. The doctor promptly cleaned me up, and he informed my mom that it should "heal up just fine," and, with time, "it may not even be noticeable." Little did I know that it would be at least a decade before my skin would completely forget this story. The scar was always a good reminder of the trials and tribulations of my body cast ... another adventure that played an important role in forming the person I am today.

A nurse at the hospital wheeled me out to the car. Dad had pulled up to the curb, and it was time for me to put weight on my atrophied legs. The wheelchair was brought right up to the front passenger side door, leaving only one step between my wheelchair and the car. "I'm not strong enough," I worried out loud.

"You can do it," my dad insisted.

While holding onto the wheelchair, I pushed myself up to a standing position. I took one step with my right leg as I let go with my arms. My father caught me as my legs collapsed, like a foal taking its first step away from its mother. He took me in his arms and gently set me in the car.

In the coming weeks, my legs were clearly uncooperative. They shook uncontrollably as I attempted to stand. Mom would often break into song: "She's got the hippy, hippy shakes." Sometimes this would make me giggle; other times it made me scream. "This isn't funny! I just want to get better! I want legs and arms like yours!" *God, I'm counting on you to get me through this! I can't do it alone and giving up is NOT an option.* I had a way of ruining a funny moment when I wanted to ... yet Mom seemed to suggest I was entitled.

In time, I got stronger ... to a point where I could walk a two-foot stretch in the living room where the oak banister became a make-shift guide bar—the kind you see in a PT clinic. I would walk back and forth hanging onto that railing as Grandma would watch me from the kitchen. "You're doing so well, Jeanie."

Grandma was such a big help to my mom during the whole ordeal. With her background as a nurse, she was able to take care of me. She slept every night on the couch in the family room. When I would yell for her to roll me over, she would rise without hesitation and run up to the base of the steps to call for my mother. "Ann. Jeanie needs to be rolled." My mom would come down just as quickly as Grandma called her.

As a kid, who thinks of this—but I truly wonder if either of them ever slept! They'd roll me over, and help me get a drink if I asked for one. Grandma would go back to the couch, and Mom would return to her bed upstairs. My mother would be up early the next morning for work. I'm sure Grandma chatted with her while I slumbered on ... I'm exhausted just thinking about it!

Grandma was more than a nurse during her stay with us. She helped me with all of my homework too. She even read to me—a novel for seventh-grade English class. We would laugh about that book for years to come, as we recalled the one thing we agreed upon—it was possibly the worst story ever written.

Before I had my cast removed, Grandma would sneak kittens into the house for me to play with when both my parents were at work. She saw me smile as a fluffy white kitten lounged on top of my cast. The little thing would meow as it walked up and down my body, as if crossing a bridge, or strolling a stretch of sidewalk. When Grandma would retrieve the kitten to take it back outside, I could feel my heart break just a little bit. Later, I might hear the scratching of claws as all five kittens tried to climb the door leading from the garage to the family room. I would wait and hope that Grandma would give in to their pleas, and appear with another kitten to entertain me for just a little longer.

My mom put a stop to this. Sneaking kittens in the house became strictly forbidden after Mom discovered that one had fleas.

She explained to the entire family, "Think how awful it will be if Jeanie gets fleas down that cast!" As much as I loved playing with the kittens, I knew that being itchy would only add to the discomfort of the cast. This was one house rule I didn't ask Grandma to break.

Once I was out of the cast, I could abandon my bed baths. Our multilevel home was still a challenge—I couldn't get up the stairs to the bathtub. However, my dad put a large construction pail in the shower stall downstairs. Mom somehow got me to the blue wheelchair in the downstairs bathroom, where she helped me remove my clothing. She would transfer me from the wheelchair to the giant overturned pail, which worked as a stable shower chair for a while.

I remember our first attempt at this. "I don't think I can do this, Mom," I declared.

"Yes, you can. And you will," she responded, turning the shower on.

An exhausting fifteen minutes later, she put me back into the wheelchair. I dried myself off and Mom helped me into my pajamas. After my hair was brushed, she wheeled me into the family room so I could rest and watch TV. In another couple of weeks, I'd be able to get myself upstairs and into a bath all on my own. That could not come soon enough.

When I finally got my cast removed, Dr. Christensen sent me home with crutches. He affirmed that they would help me learn to walk again—like I was a toddler learning this skill for the first time. The idea of crutches scared me more than anyone knew. I hemmed and hawed about them, and told my parents, "I don't think they'll work. I guess I can keep practicing while holding onto the banister." My brother Tom must have been listening to this conversation because the next thing I knew, he had the crutches in his hands.

"Jean, you can do this. Just watch me," he said, placing the crutches under his arms. Then the foolishness began. He walked with the crutches as if he had noodles for legs. Like Charlie Chaplin, he was all over the family room pretending to fall to the left and then to the right. Just as his legs looked like they would give out, he popped up, and the foolishness started again. He swung one crutch to the left and then the other crutch to the right. He was practically dancing. Meanwhile, Mom and I were laughing uncontrollably. (This might have been one of those times when laughter caused some embarrassment. Unlike Pavlov's dog, I never salivated. *My* conditioned response was wet pants!)

Tom must have sensed success at this point, because he suddenly stopped the whole production. "Here you go," he said, holding out the crutches.

I took them, and with a big smile, I stood up from my chair, relieved that I was wearing a bladder control pad. I hadn't come this far to never walk again. I could at least show my brother my best try.

A Full Day

I OPENED MY EYES AND MY PINK CLOCK RADIO READ 6:10 A.M.
I must have been the only eighth grader in the history of the world
who didn't really need an alarm. I have never slept long enough to
hear the thing go off. But it was habit to set it. So I silenced the
alarm before it had a chance to go off, then climbed out of bed. I
grabbed my Guess jeans and a purple sweatshirt, also branded with
"Guess"—but in this case the trademark was spelled out in a rainbow of colors.

I dropped to the ground in order to slide my legs, one at a time,
into the expensive jeans. I leaned back on my shoulders to lift my
butt off the floor, then pulled the jeans up to my waist. I buttoned
the pants before I sat up to tackle the shirt, which slid over my head
and shoulders with ease. I wondered how it would feel to dress
standing up—like the girls did in the locker room at Fred Moore
Junior High. I never understood how they could do that—stand
without losing their balance, with arms, neck, and head lost in a
bulky sweater. Or, how they could put a shoe on without even sitting down, balanced like a ballerina, sliding toes and heel in almost
simultaneously. Amazing feats of agility were accomplished every
day in my junior high, while I watched and knew that I would certainly never be an upright dresser—and that was okay with me. I
still got downstairs in record time before breakfast.

After a bowl of Life cereal, I grabbed the phonebook from the
bottom shelf of the end table and placed it strategically on the floor

behind the couch. I turned the television on to *Bewitched*, my morning program of choice. This was an old show, in syndication on one of the cable networks. Not my favorite sitcom, but Darrin and Sam entertained me for twenty minutes while I stretched my calves using the thick Minneapolis phone book. I walked back behind the couch, stepped onto the five-inch-thick book, my toes on the top and my heels hitting the plush carpet. The slight burn in my calves felt like a Christmas gift to me. This part of my daily routine was not by choice—standard procedure if I intended to maintain any control over my walking throughout the day. By this age, I had grown compliant and eager to do what was needed to safeguard my mobility.

Of course, I was still a toe-walker. And if I wasn't tippy-toeing around the house, I could be found dragging my feet across the floor, leaving deep rub marks on my Reebok sneakers. Yet, my stretches had brought me a long way from the year I was seven and we visited Disney World on a family trip. That was the time I dragged my toes along the Magic Kingdom grounds so heavily that I not only wore holes through my sneakers, but my new white socks were shredded.

My twenty-minute stretches were finished before Sam could even make peace between Endora and Darrin. I hopped off the "book that gets used" and put it back on its shelf.

I climbed the stairs and knocked on the bathroom door just outside my bedroom. Mom opened it, standing in her usual pose— a curling iron in one hand, and a comb in the other.

"Can you put a clip in my hair?" I asked, holding up the metal barrette.

"Sure."

I followed her into her dark bedroom and took a seat on the floor at the foot of the bed. She sat on the edge of the mattress and began to brush my hair. Dad was still curled up in the blankets, trying to get his last bit of sleep before a long, physical day of work. With silent precision, Mom once again placed my barrette like a professional stylist—in the dark, and in record time. I smiled, and whispered, "Thanks," then bounced into my own room to tackle my bangs.

My curling iron was hot and ready for me to attempt to make

my bangs as big as I possibly could. I took the top clumps of hair, curled them *back*, and sprayed them with the potent Aqua Net. Then I clasped the bottom half of my bangs, curled them *under*, and showered them with Aqua Net as well. I ratted and teased and added even more hair spray in hopes of getting the look that all the popular girls had at school. Thick clouds of hair spray polluted my room. It's a wonder I could see my reflection in the mirror, or breathe without coughing. *Rats—another bad hair day.* I would have to settle for limp curls, drooping in my face. *Just once I want hair like Alyssa Milano from Who's the Boss?*

"Ready?" Mom asked as she grabbed her car keys.

"Yep." Once I pulled on a jacket, I grabbed my book bag and my clarinet case, and we were off in Mom's black Ford Taurus.

My mother dropped me at school every day on her way to work. As she pulled up to one of the largest junior highs in Minnesota, I climbed out to the curb and slammed the door. I knew this was when the real part of the day began, and I was on my own in the world of not-so-nice kids. This day, like most, would end in complete exhaustion.

I dropped my clarinet off in the band room and kept moving as smoothly as possible. I trudged through the crowded hallway to locker number one, where I hung my book bag and jacket. Not too many kids knew that I actually had two lockers. Mr. Halloway, my guidance counselor, wanted to simplify logistics for me as I navigated this incredibly large school. He arranged for me to have lockers on the first and third floors. I could divide my books up and store them closest to each classroom. Since there were seven periods in the day, this helped me avoid tardies. Mr. Halloway also arranged to have me leave each of my classes five minutes early to avoid the crowded hallways. This made the start of every new semester a little awkward since students would stare as I stood up to leave early from class. But they figured it out, and after a week or so, no one even seemed to notice.

Mr. Halloway also arranged it so I could keep a set of textbooks at home and a set of the same books at school, so I didn't have to carry forty pounds of books home from the bus stop after school. I don't think too many of the kids knew this secret either. Between my parents' requests and Mr. Halloway's help, junior high was probably a lot less stressful than it might have been. Yet, the potential for disaster seemed to hover in the air around all these morphing adolescents.

I arrived at home economics, my first-period class, trying to mentally prepare for our cooking unit. I hated cooking. It didn't help that I lacked the dexterity to lift heavy ingredients like sacks of flour … or pour liquids to a precise line … or measure dry spices with Barbie doll-sized spoons.

I remember the day we made pancakes. The classroom began filling up with eighth graders—mostly hormones and fragile egos. I recall feeling lucky when kitchen groups were assigned because the kids in my group were kind to me. I washed my hands and fumbled with my apron tie until someone helped me secure it around my small waist. The teacher delivered the written pancake recipe to each group, and we had forty-five minutes to cook, eat, and clean up.

More than anything, I wanted to cook like the other kids in class. I wanted to mix and pour with ease and grace. Since this was the first class of the day, my body seemed more cooperative than usual. Call it adrenaline or keen senses that come when faced with something new, I suddenly felt lucky to have the energy and dexterity to whip up a successful pancake batter! While some classmates dropped their breakfast on the floor, my pancakes turned out near-perfect that day … beyond the expectations of thirteen-year-olds, anyway. I scored big with my kitchen-mates.

Class was nearly over, so I put my apron in the laundry basket, washed my hands, and picked up my books. Talk about an efficient breakfast—I still left the class five minutes early for my trek to second period. If anyone noticed, they didn't make a big deal of it. We were well into the quarter, and they were all used to my early exits by now.

The first day of every quarter, I stressed out about telling each teacher of my "arrangement" to leave class early. Some of them looked at me like I was trying to get away with something. Others seemed accepting, probably because they had observed my struggles through the halls to reach my next class. To appease the skeptics, I came armed with a "hall pass" from Mr. Halloway. This little yellow piece of paper simply stated that "Jean Sharon has permission to leave class five minutes early." This sort of pass was usually reserved for students with broken arms or legs—a temporary condition. With a look that seemed to say, "Will this be going on indefinitely? Or are you going to heal like the rest of them?" the skeptics reluctantly accepted my pass, and ignored my early departures.

Mornings flew by, and by the end of fourth period, Mr. Mueller's science class, I actually scooted out a full ten minutes early. The additional five minutes allowed for a side trip to the nurse's office where I took my prescribed three and one-half baclofen pills promptly at twelve o'clock. Mr. Mueller was *not* happy about my early departure. Apparently one of the *skeptics*, Mr. Mueller believed I was scheming for an extended lunch.

I stood up from my desk and began making my way toward the door.

"Where are you going, Jean?" he questioned, his black, bushy eyebrows frowned in disapproval.

Here we go again. I endured his routine questioning every few weeks. *For a science teacher, you have a lousy memory.*

"I'm going to the nurse's office and then to lunch," I replied.

I left the classroom as gracefully as my legs would allow, without looking back for his permission. I was certain that he stood outside the classroom door watching me walk away. I sensed his eyes on my back, but I didn't bother to turn around. *He must see me struggling to walk. What is his problem?* No doubt he watched to make sure that I did not veer from a direct path to the nurse's office.

When I turned the corner, I knew I was in the clear—not that I was trying to get away with something. Yet I felt kind of like a tough kid, walking away from the teacher like that. *I bet the cool kids were surprised that "Goody Two-shoes" Jean snubbed the teacher.* I felt superior for the moment, but deep down Mr. Mueller made me so nervous. I was a rule-follower, and he doubted me. Some weeks later, I learned that my mom gave the school a call about his harassment. *Hmm ... I wondered why Mr. Mueller suddenly stopped bugging me.*

My body knew that it was lunchtime as I pushed the solid glass door to leave the nurse's office. By this time of the day, I struggled to take every step as I walked past the rooms full of activity, to descend the stairs to the cafeteria. The smell of greasy tater tots and chicken made my stomach growl. One advantage to early arrival: I could carry my tray to a nearby empty table before hundreds of hungry kids arrived.

I ate and nervously looked out of the corners of my eyes to see who of my friends would join me first. I hated sitting alone for those few minutes. I felt as if everyone checked in on me, thinking, "The loser is sitting by herself again."

Traci walked up to me with her tray in hand. *Finally.* She sat down and I felt instant relief. Her shoulder-length blonde hair was in a clip similar to mine ... except she had clearly dodged the curling iron problems that I experienced that morning. Her blue eyes, slightly hidden by her glasses, grew with concern as I told her about the incident with Mr. Mueller. Then, a boy from the ninth grade abruptly interrupted my story.

"Do you want this drug?" he asked, holding out his hand to show a brown pill.

Traci quickly replied, "No." He looked directly at me.

I rolled my eyes to inform him that I was no dummy. "It's ibuprofen!" I stated with a scowl, and he walked away.

I breathed a sigh of relief, and Traci and I continued to talk and laugh about the day's events as we finished our mundane meals. It was time for me to start my stroll to the next class, but I would need to make a pit stop at locker number two first.

I despised this floor of my building. Yet, these ugly orange lockers in fact helped me keep my balance as I glided my right hand across the surface of them while navigating the hallway. My off-kilter balance actually reminded me that at least my stiff legs and heel cords would get me where I needed to go, if I just took time to concentrate. *My limp's slowing me down today ... my right knee is throbbing worse than yesterday.*

I thought about stopping in the bathroom before the next class, but pushed that consideration out of mind almost as fast as it had entered. I never used a school restroom—too much effort to pull my pants down and up again. I was already leaving class early. I'd hold my pee all day before I'd ask a teacher to forgive a tardy due to a potty stop.

With spastic diplegia, I had never experienced leg pain until shortly after I got out of my body cast. My walk had changed. My knees no longer knocked one another, but because of the abnormal walk, and likely due to the surgical cuts made to alter things internally, knee pressure surged as the day moved on. *No doubt it hurts more now because my walk gets worse with the day. But I don't know how to move any differently.*

I reached the stairs. I stopped at the base and looked up the wide stairwell. I placed my left foot on the far left side of the bottom step. *Take a breath ... now lift the right leg onto the bottom step.* As soon as it was stable on the step, I raised my left leg to the next step. Methodical, like primitive robot commands—*lift, then step ... lift, then step*—I wasn't able to race up the steps like all of the other kids who frequently passed me as they sprinted to the top of a flight of stairs.

Not all of the stairs went from the basement to the third floor. *This sucks! I'm thirteen years old and even I know that this school has a stupid setup.* This particular stairway, for instance, only brought me to the first floor. I would have to navigate another long corridor to find a different flight of stairs that led to the second floor. Most buildings were not compliant with ADA policies yet. *This is ridiculous—why don't we have an elevator!?* This thought bubble popped into my head every day at this same moment.

As soon as I reached the top step, I could see one of the ninth-grade science teachers—one I never had, with the salt-and-pepper hair.

"Hello, Jean," he stated with a smile. "How's your day going?"

He says hello to me and asks me how I'm doing every day. I smile back.

"Oh, it's good." I am grateful for his greeting—I can count on his friendly inquiry, and he never questioned whether I was supposed to be in the hallway or not. I believe he had a general understanding of my situation—and that's all he needed to know to lighten my day.

I entered Mr. Copeland's empty social studies classroom, opened the closet door at the front of the room, and bent down to grab my heavy textbook. The brown book cover had hearts drawn all over it—my trademark, although no other students put their books in there.

At the end of the very first class day with Mr. Copeland, I had watched with a puzzled look as he abruptly snatched my textbook back from me, and placed it in the closet. He then lightly tapped the base of the closet door with his dress shoe.

"You can keep your book in here, Jean. It's too heavy to be lugging all the way to your locker," he said. His beard did not camouflage his kind expression.

My heart filled with hope and I smiled back at him. "Oh, and tell your brother Mike 'Hi.'" I didn't have a chance to reply since he quickly followed with, "And let him know, it's clear who got the looks in the family—it's not him."

My smile broadened. I would be more than thrilled to deliver that message to Mike.

Mike had told me how much he enjoyed Mr. Copeland's class. He had warned me that he was not an easy teacher, but that he was really nice and liked to joke around. I could see that my brother was right.

On this particular day, I pulled my heavy book out of the closet, took it to my seat in the back, and sat down to rest my eyes. I would have only a moment before the other eighth graders came pouring into the room. *If I rest just a little bit, I'll be way more productive.* Even holding a pencil became a challenge by this time of the day, and Mr. Copeland's notes on the board might be easier to copy if I took a time-out from the stress of this full day.

The bell rang, and I had to admit—Mr. Copeland's map of the Middle East didn't really hook me. He tried his best, I'm sure, but like most junior high schoolers, I retained only a vague idea of the Persian Gulf's importance … something about oil. I glanced at the clock and remembered I had gym next. I was especially concerned with leaving five minutes early on phys ed days. *If I don't leave on time, there is no way that I will make it down to the pool for swimming.*

Once the clock indicated my time to leave, I got up, returned my book to the closet, and headed out into the hall. I stopped back at my locker on the first floor, just outside the office, and grabbed my school bag and jacket. *When gym is over I won't have time to come back to get my stuff before I get on the bus.* I stuffed my coat into my Esprit bag and walked as fast as I could down to the basement. Luckily for me, my knee didn't bother me going *down* the stairs.

I made it into the girls' locker room near the pool. I absolutely hated these swimming classes. It was bad enough changing for phys ed when I didn't have to take my bra and underwear off. My friends Rebecca, Stacy, and Rachel were getting into their suits at the same time. I was looking about as uncomfortable as I felt. Getting dressed was a challenge for me in the privacy of my own bedroom. The added stress of changing in front of these girls, plus knowing I had to be in the pool area in less than five minutes, made my arms and legs stiffen up.

I'm not sure if I'll be able to do this. I lost my balance just before I pulled my suit up. I heard the "slap" of my butt cheeks hit the wooden bench and my face filled with embarrassment. Rebecca laughed as her big blue eyes smiled at me. I knew that she was not laughing at me, but laughing with me. I could trust her for that.

I stood up quickly, took off my bra, and instantly covered my breasts with my blue swimsuit. I really didn't think that we had swimming lessons at school to teach us how to swim, but rather, to break us in for other humiliations to come in life.

Mrs. Lutz instructed all of the kids to get in the pool. I walked over to the other side to find Kyle, my special phys ed teacher who was young, fit, and a great swimmer. Today he was dressed in jeans and a shirt. *He's not getting in the pool with me today.* I tried not to show my disappointment. Last year Kyle got in the water with me, but this year he didn't. He never really told me why he wouldn't get in the water with me anymore. My mom said, "It's probably because you're older now ... probably not appropriate for him to be in the water with you."

As I stepped into the pool using the ladder, my muscles tensed up even more. *I can't catch a break today.* I often thought, *It's not exactly easy for me to stand on solid ground ... so let's put me in a pool with a bunch of crazy kids!* The wave action caused by all the swimmers was wild. *If I'm lucky I can bob just often enough to catch a breath.*

Despite my sarcasm, once I talked to Kyle, I always happily resigned myself to do what he asked—he was a great teacher. Fun yet cautious, he never asked me to do things that he knew I couldn't do, unlike other special-ed teachers I had in the past. Kyle must have been a good listener because he never seemed to forget my fears, my likes, my dislikes ... he understood and accepted my reservations when I had them. *I only have to do this for thirty minutes and then I can go home.* He understood that I didn't feel comfortable in the pool all alone, and taught with an empathetic approach to everything.

"Here, you grab onto this," he said to me as he put the end of a pole into the water. *I've never seen one of these before. It kind of looks like my dad's fishing net. Except, instead of a net, there is a rubbery handle for me to hold onto.*

"You're gonna work on your back float today," Kyle informed me.

I would give it my best—*at least I have this pole to hang onto.* It helped that I trusted Kyle. I didn't trust a lot of people when I was in the water—only my mom and dad. I worked steadily on the back float, and then Kyle told me it was okay to get out of the pool.

"You did a good job today. Go get dressed and head for the bus," he said with a smile. Why would I argue with a few extra minutes to undress before the locker room overflowed with students again? I toweled off as I walked briskly away from the pool.

But, Mrs. Lutz stopped me just before I opened the locker room door.

"Where are you going?"

"I'm getting dressed," I said.

"It's too early," she scowled. "There's fifteen minutes of class left. You need to get back in the pool."

Kyle politely explained to her, "It takes Jean longer than the other kids to get changed out of a wet swimsuit." I could tell by the look in her eyes, Mrs. Lutz was not buying it. *Wow, he understands my struggle with wet spandex better than she does? What's wrong with this woman?*

Unable to win this battle, Kyle gave me a look that said I had to go back into the pool. With tears stinging my eyes, I reluctantly climbed back in the water. But I wasn't thinking about swimming. My mind reeled with the worries of changing from wet suit to dry clothes in minutes, then boarding my bus before all of the other students flooded the hallways. *God, please keep me strong. Please, don't let me break out in tears!*

This stress magnified my spasticity. Kyle must have seen it. I got the feeling he knew that I was scared. "Jean, get out of the pool. That's enough for today." In the pool, out of the pool—talk about heightening my anxiety! But I listened to Kyle once again, and headed for the locker room.

Once my swimsuit was off, I dried my body with my towel and put my legs through my white underwear. Before I pulled up my panties, I placed a Kotex pad adhesive down. *I've got my period. No wonder my stiffness is worse today.* My period made everything more difficult—not just inconvenient, but more spastic.

I placed my bra around my rib cage and hooked it in the front. I tried to turn it around, but I couldn't. I must not have dried off completely. The combination of wet skin and my anxious grip made it impossible to rotate the cups to the front so I could slip my arms through each strap. *What am I going to do? If I don't get dressed on time, I'll never make it to my bus.* No matter how hard I tried, my bra wouldn't rotate. I moved on to my jeans. *I'll go back to my bra after my jeans, socks, and shoes are on. Maybe my back will be dry enough and I'll be able to turn it around.*

I was dressed from the waist down, but I still couldn't twist my bra. I glanced at the clock on the wall. *I should be walking out to the bus right now!*

Panic consumed my body and I suddenly understood what pa-ralysis felt like. My eyes filled with tears. *Don't cry! I'd rather drown in the school pool than have the other girls see me cry.* At that moment, girls began flooding the locker room, stripping out of their wet suits, and changing into their clothes to go home.

One of the swimmers, Sarah, turned to me and asked, "What's wrong?"

"I can't get my bra on," I whispered under my breath.

"Let me help," she whispered back. And without looking for my approval, she quickly turned my bra around, like it was her own. While I slipped each arm through the straps, Sarah reached for my sweatshirt and guided it over my head. Then she led my arms, one at a time, through the sweatshirt sleeves, like a hired caregiver. She never said another word as we both grabbed our bags of belongings to race out the door. Fixated on not missing the bus, and out of breath from rushing, I never even thanked her.

Sarah helped me that day in a way that none of the other kids had before. Although we were classmates from elementary school, we weren't exactly close friends. Yet, Sarah had always been really nice to me—she had such a kind nature. God had given her the gifts of nurturing, understanding, and acceptance and somehow I was blessed to have her in my life.

I hobbled up the stairs as fast as I could. *I just have to deal with the pain piercing through my knee. I have to make this bus!* I opened the door that led me outside, and the bell rang, signaling the end of a full school day. Kids poured out of the doors, and although the sidewalk was slick from snow that day, my bus was luckily parked near this closest exit. *What a relief.*

I gripped the handle and leveraged my way up the steep bus entrance. I spotted an empty seat, not too far down the left side of the isle. *Ah, thirty minutes of rest—that is, if people leave me alone.* I pulled out a book to read, hoping that the other kids would ignore me. The bus ride home was one the worst parts of my day—mostly due to two younger girls; I think they were in the class behind me. For some reason, they enjoyed imitating me, or saying mean things behind my back … just loud enough for me to hear. On this particular day, I was spared. Everyone left me alone.

When the bus reached my stop, I marched down the three large steps, carrying my clarinet. Chad, a ninth grader, always got off at the same stop as me. He was with a friend, and they both slowly walked ahead of me. Chad stopped and turned. Indicating my clarinet case, "Here, let me carry that for you."

With two and a half blocks left to walk, which felt like a mile on days like these, I was very grateful.

"Thanks," I said, handing over the case to him. I was exhausted and knew it would take all my energy to walk home with some degree of dignity. Chad and his friend hiked slower than they needed to, keeping some small talk going along the way. As we reached the part of the road where we needed to separate to go to our respective houses, he handed my clarinet back to me, and asked if I would be able to carry my case the rest of the way home.

"Yes, I can get it. Thanks," I answered.

"No problem," he said. "Have a good night."

I reached my home after walking another ten minutes—about half a block. I opened the door, stepped onto the dark linoleum, and made a crash-landing on my hands and knees. I yanked off my Reebok tennis shoes and sprinted clumsily into the bathroom, which I desperately needed to use.

The closer I got to the toilet, the more I felt the urge to pee. *My bladder can't hold an entire day's worth of liquid much longer.* I undid my pants, but I could tell it was going to be a struggle to get them down. I sidestepped to the vanity, and leaned my butt against the sink. Using the edge of the vanity and my spastic-tight hands, I began to shimmy my pants down. Gaining about a half-inch with each pull, I jerked my jeans down far enough after a few dozen tugs. *Halleluiah! No mess ... I haven't wet my pants this time!* I wasn't surprised, since I hadn't had much to laugh about today. If I had wet my pants, laughing would have been the cause of it.

I stood, desperately trying to yank my jeans back up in one fluid pull. *Not gonna happen. I should know better.* My cotton panties move pretty easily, but pulling my jeans up is harder than getting them down. *Why would today be any different?* Again, I sidestepped and leaned against the vanity for extra leverage in order to perform my routine of tug, pull, tug, pull until my tight-fisted grip shimmied my pants up and over my hips. I parked these experiences deep inside my memory—a constant reminder that I should *not* try a bathroom break at school. An exploding bladder in the privacy of my own home was one thing … in a junior high restroom stall it would be quite another.

I strolled into the kitchen to grab some Cheez-Its. *I'm so hungry.* Food was just what I needed to help take the tightness out of my arms and legs. I decided to bring the entire box of crackers with me to my parents' bedroom to watch thirty minutes of television. When I heard the door open, I knew Mom was home from work. I hiked down to the kitchen, sat at the counter, and began doing my math homework while she dished up dinner—something easy to warm up since I had church class that night. *I really don't want to go to church class. It would be really nice to stay home and watch TV.* A girl can dream, right?

By 5:30 P.M., I found myself at Saint Patrick's Church with kids who were not all that nice. For starters, I didn't go to the same school as most of them, so no one talked to me. I eased into a chair, watching and listening as they laughed and clearly had fun with one another. That's when Trent, the one kid who *did* go to my school, stood up and said, "This is how Jean walks."

I looked over to find him strutting across the room, his lanky legs turned inwards, his knees almost hitting one another. His left arm was bent up to his chest as he limped around the table where most of the kids were sitting.

I felt tears welling up. *I can't let him or anyone else in this room see me cry.* I looked away from him, opened my religious-ed book, and pretended to read the pages. *He won't get a response from me tonight. I don't have the energy left today, and he's not worth it anyway. At any moment, the teacher will walk in, and he'll quit. Then Mom picks me up at seven.* The clock hands could not move fast enough.

By 7:30 P.M., Mom and I were back home.

"You need to take your bath, Jean."

I don't think I have enough energy left in me to do this. But I carried my pajamas and clean underwear to my bed so they were within easy reach after my bath. I turned the faucet on, adjusted the temp of the water, then slid onto the toilet to rally enough energy to tug and pull my jeans off for the last time today. I got them down to my ankles more easily than expected, but that was where it stopped. I couldn't lift my right foot, even an inch off of the ground, to pull my leg out of the jeans. I tried three times—then ... *That's it!*

"Other people just do things!" I screamed at the top of my lungs. *All I want to do is take these stupid pants off and get into this stupid tub so I can get my pajamas on and be done with this stupid day!*

My mom heard me yell. She was on the other side of the door before I even finished my thoughts of frustration.

"Do you need help?" she asked. I suddenly felt like a thirteen-year-old baby.

I would love more than anything to tell her, "No, I can do it." But the fact is, I can't. I need help. I'm thirteen years old and I need help taking my pants off. No other students at Fred Moore School need their Moms to help them take a bath tonight.

"Yes," I answered. "I need your help getting my pants off."

My mom slowly opened the door to see me with tears in my eyes. She was one of the only people that I ever allowed to see my tears. I knew that she wouldn't judge me for what I was able or not able to do. She just helped me do what I couldn't on my own, and pushed me to do the things she knew I could handle.

She stepped into the bathroom, closed the door, then knelt down beside me. Gently, she guided one leg at a time. Without saying a word, she grabbed the bottom of my sweatshirt and pulled it up and over my head.

"Trent imitated my walk at church tonight," I blurted, with tears spilling down my cheeks. "Why would he do that? And of all places, at church!"

Mom focused on folding my jeans and said, "Some kids can only make themselves feel better by putting others down." Looking up, she advised, "Don't worry about it."

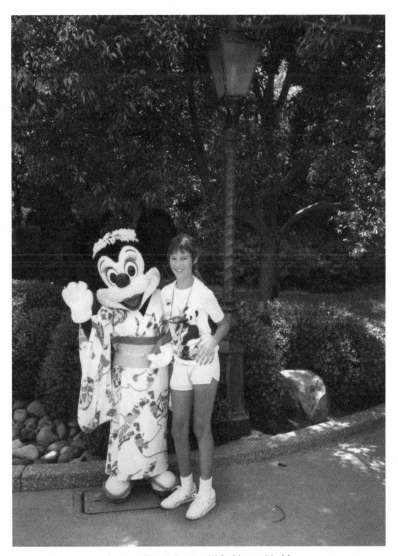

Jean at Epcot Center, Walt Disney World

She stood up, ready to close the door. "Sit in the tub for a while. That'll relax your muscles."

After a good long soak, I pulled the drain, rolled onto my side, then onto all fours so I could secure my balance before standing up.

The spasms began just in time for me to step out of the tub. I waited a moment before grabbing my towel, then stepped onto the light-blue bathmat that I helped Mom pick out a few years ago. I slowly wrapped the towel around me.

Out of the tub ... time to fight my way into my pajamas. I will do this without help tonight.

Once in my pajamas, I eased down to Mom and Dad's bedroom floor to watch TV. I pulled myself up promptly at 9:00 P.M., said goodnight to Dad, and headed for my own room. My mom followed behind me.

Positioned flat on my back in bed, I let Mom stand above me as she extended my left leg under her right shoulder for my usual bedtime stretch. "This is really tight tonight," she informed me. I nodded in agreement.

She stretched both of my hamstrings and both of my heel cords. The welcome burning in my muscles brought relief to this full day in ways I could not articulate, to Mom or to anyone.

"How's that?" she asked.

"Good." I think I sounded grateful.

As I rolled onto my stomach, ready for some serious sleep, I felt my arms and legs tense up. The muscle spasms always felt the most intense just before sleep. *This is going to be a twenty- or thirty-minute session, I can tell.* My muscles would calm when they were good and ready. There was nothing Mom or I could do to stop my spastic muscles when they started up like this. Strong-willed and uncooperative, they took over ... all I could do was wait it out.

"Here, let me help you," Mom said, pulling my leg braces into place. I was weak and annoyed by the spasms, so rather than fight it, I asked, "Can you rub my back?"

"Sure," she answered, taking a seat on the edge of my bed.

She placed her hand under my pajama shirt. Her fingernails went up and down my back in a very slow, predictable manner that helped my muscles relax. Five minutes would do it—I was feeling better, and ready to sleep. "How's that? See you in the morning," she said, thinking she was done with massage therapy for the night.

"Can you rub my head too?"

"Just for a couple minutes," she smiled.

After a few minutes of massaging my head, Mom stepped away from my bed and walked to my door. She turned to say, "Goodnight, Jean."

"Goodnight."

She shut off the light and gently closed the door. It seems unfair that after all of her efforts, my body still jumped into full spasm. Yet, it wasn't a big surprise to me. I just remained calm and let the spasms take over my body. After a tiring day, this was completely expected. The muscles wouldn't stop tightening up, so I kicked into a special breathing that I found to be helpful. If anyone outside of my family ever saw me do this, they'd think I was in labor. It reminded me of those movie scenes where the pregnant woman breaks into Lamaze breathing just before the baby pops out with that newborn cry.

"He, he, hoo. He, he, hoo." Of course, I wouldn't feel the joy of a tiny, swaddled infant in my arms once the deep breathing stopped. The best I could hope for was a spasm-less night's sleep until my alarm clock read 6:10 A.M.—time for another crazy day at Fred Moore Junior High. I have to admit, some days I felt trapped in Bill Murray's *Groundhog Day* pattern. *If life could just be a little less full tomorrow ...* this was my last thought as my silly breathing faded and I drifted off to sleep.

My Movie-Poster Soul Mate

WITH COACHING FROM MOM, AND MINOR SUCCESS IN THE home-ec kitchen at school, I decided it was time to do some of my own cooking. *If I can help Mom chop vegetables or mix ingredients, I should be able to make my own meal.* But what culinary tasks can be completed without *standing*? Who stirs, pours, and pops pans into an oven from a sitting position?

Standing for long periods of time was my nemesis. I felt insecure, off-balance, and rather unsafe over a hot stove. Plus, my legs tired easily. So, what dish could be completed in a short time span? My favorite, of course—Kraft Macaroni and Cheese! So, once a week during the summer, I started my new ritual of boiling noodles, then adding butter, milk, and that scrumptious cheese powder, to create the best mac and cheese dinner ever.

On one particular Friday afternoon, I was a bit weak and spastic. I really craved mac and cheese, and felt ready for the challenge to transform this box of dry ingredients into a meal. Just when I added the noodles to the boiling water, I suddenly lost my balance. I found myself taking four steps backward, faster than I knew I could. My back hit the counter and, as hard as I tried to maintain my balance, my legs gradually gave out on me. I lost all control of my body. I began sliding slowly down toward the floor with my shoulders up against the cupboards adjacent to the stove. When my butt hit the ground, I growled with frustration. *Klutz! What now?*

I allowed myself to sit on the brown linoleum floor for a minute to cool down before I attempted to rescue myself, and get back to cooking. I looked up at the pan of hot steam on the stove, and heard the rolling rumble of water. Instantly I realized, *I've got to pull myself up and stir those noodles. Those buggers are gonna boil over!*

I leaned forward. My body was stuck to the cupboard. Literally, I was attached! ... like sticky noodles glued to the bottom of the pan those times when I couldn't stir often or fast enough. When I slid down to the floor, the back of my bra apparently looped through the vertical handle of the lower kitchen cupboard door. *What in the world? I'm hooked!*

I was not only hooked, I was mad! I pulled myself forward again—this time with a little more authority—only to have the cupboard door open an inch. I tried to stand straight up without leaning forward, even though I had never been able to tackle such a feat. *Nothing!* I didn't have the quad strength to make a vertical move to a standing position. I leaned forward again, but the cupboard opened again.

"Aghhhhhhhhhhhhhhh!" I couldn't help but scream with frustration. "Other people just do things! Why can't I be like them, God?"

I kept trying to pull myself forward with no luck whatsoever. I peered up at the handle of the steaming, bubbling pan and began to panic. *If that boils over, I'll be showered by scalding hot water.* I had enough minor burns in my life to know I needed to think fast.

I have to get my bra off. I'm not sure how, but that's the fastest way to get unhooked. Clearly, I had to remove my shirt and bra to avoid a 911 call. The modest teenager in me quickly weighed the embarrassment of being discovered in my bra on the kitchen floor vs. potential second-degree burns. (Yes, I had paid attention in home-ec class!) *What if my dad comes home? Or worse yet, what if one of his employees walks into the house—their paychecks are sitting right on the kitchen table.* Today was payday for Dad's workers, and we had an open door policy for all his men.

As fast as my spastic grip allowed me, I ripped off my peach tank top and leaned forward one more time. My bra popped loose from the cupboard. I lunged forward from the release, and on my hands and knees, scrambled to pull my tank back on. I took a deep breath, leaned forward, stood long enough to feel my balance, then drained my noodles. *This better taste good.*

* * *

My clock read 5:30 A.M. This was early, even for me on a school day, but my hours had changed since I left Fred Moore Junior High and entered high school. I leaned across my bed to turn on my lamp, which illuminated Johnny Depp's subtle smile. *People* magazine eventually named him "Sexiest Man Alive"—twice—and I have always wondered why it took so long. His dark brown eyes, olive skin, and a smile that would melt any teenage girl's heart camouflaged the fact that he was almost twice my age.

My focus shifted from the alarm clock to the ninety-nine photos of him checkerboarding my bedroom wall. Contrary to what Tom always said, *I am not obsessed.* I defended my Johnny Depp fascination by scolding Tom with, "He's a fantastic actor! If you watched *Edward Scissorhands* once, you'd realize this." Actually, before *Edward Scissorhands*, I had no idea who Johnny Depp was. But as I watched him speak, his eyes on the big screen hypnotizing me, I knew I was hooked! I remember when my friend Amy set me straight.

"Who is this guy?" I swooned.

"That's Johnny Depp," Amy replied in a matter-of-fact tone.

"Who?"

I had never heard the name before, but tuned in to *21 Jump Street* after viewing *Edward Scissorhands*—and that's when I made up my mind. My room was going to be wallpapered with that face. I didn't care how many *Tiger Beat* magazines I had to buy, or posters I needed to purchase—I would fulfill my dream. And that's how I wound up opening my eyes every morning to Johnny Depp: *Benny and Joon, What's Eating Gilbert Grape, Cry-Baby, Edward Scissorhands* ... two big *21 Jump Street* posters. I added an array of magazine eight-by-tens, and covered every inch of wall space.

I found myself spending a lot of time in my room, gazing at Johnny, and praying for the day when I could tell him what a brilliant actor he was ... even if my brother insisted Johnny was only "a little guy with arms that aren't strong enough to hold the gun he uses on *21 Jump Street*."

I turned my boom box on to KDWB and slowly got dressed. In the family room, I performed my heel-cord stretches—my morning ritual for the past ten years. *If this is what it takes to keep me out of a wheelchair* ... It was actually relaxing—good downtime, like yoga, I suppose. Years later, with spasticity gone and my muscles operating *without* this stretch, I would remind myself of this insight.

At fifteen, although a high school student, I still had to ride the bus. It would be another year before I could even think about taking a driver's test. In the winter, I found myself walking to my bus stop in the 6:20 A.M. darkness. The street I lived on didn't have any lampposts, so I was at the mercy of our porch light, which guided me like a lighthouse beacon all the way to the end of our driveway. The bright Minnesota snow led me the rest of the way. After a five-minute wait in the sub-zero-degree air, my bus pulled up. I carefully climbed the three steps, smiled, and greeted my bus driver, who resembled Jolly Old St. Nicholas. *Seriously, this song goes off in my head every day ... if he only knew ... but then he might shave his white beard off.* I refrained from humming the tune.

"Good morning!" he cheerfully greeted me.

Jolly Old Saint Nicholas ...

"Hello," I replied. Who couldn't smile with Christmas sounding off in your head every day?

I was the first stop on St. Nick's fifty-minute route. Unlike every other bus driver I'd had in the past decade, this pleasant man tuned the radio to KDWB, a station many of his riders preferred. It made taking the bus more tolerable for teens counting down to DMV Day, and created a cool-grandpa image for him.

I sat alone for much of the ride. It was far too dark to read, so I listened to Dave Ryan on the radio, bantering between tunes. Bryan Adams's "I Do It for You," (clearly overplayed), reminded me of a movie I had never seen—*Robin Hood, Prince of Thieves*. Karen, another bus-riding tenth grader, stated that it reminded her of her boyfriend.

"It was our song ... before we broke up," she shared with heavy melancholy in her voice.

Long pause.

"What?" she finally asked, a bit defensive and obviously concerned with my reaction to this private news.

"That's so sad," I said, quickly covering the real question that popped into my mind: *What in the world is she talking about? How would I know what it's like to have a "song," much less a "boyfriend"?*

The guys at school weren't interested in hanging out with me. One thing I counted on—I would never have a boyfriend. I envisioned being the "favorite" aunt, simply because guys don't swoon over girls like me. This too was part of God's plan and I slowly grew accustomed to the idea.

Nevertheless, I felt at ease in Blaine High School. It was as if the past three years at Fred Moore never happened. Most of those Fred Moore classmates enrolled in Anoka High School. I, on the other hand, went to Blaine, where the students were so much easier to be around. In the first two months at my new school, I hadn't been made fun of once. Not even a stare! It was as though all the Blaine kids had someone at home just like me. I don't even think they said things behind my back. In fact, when we had collaborative projects, students who barely knew my name approached me.

"Hey, wanna be partners?" It was so nice not to have to search with that rather pleading look on my face, "Please ask me to join you." I hated pity, but I despised begging even more. As if I were asking my peers, *Come on, dig deep enough to do the right thing. Don't let the cripple stand here alone, all forlorn, without a partner ...* The last thing I wanted to do was guilt someone into working with me.

Even more impressive, the Blaine juniors and seniors talked to me the most! I began thinking, *I don't really know people in my own grade. What will I do next year when the seniors graduate and I don't have them to rely on any longer?*

* * *

My first period of the day was phys ed, and Kyle continued on as my gym teacher. The previous week, my class was completing a volleyball unit, so Kyle had taken me to the computer room, where we played golf. I wasn't sure what he had up his sleeve this time.

"Hey, Jean. What do you think of this? I want you to consider taking the weight lifting class." He explained that it would be great for strengthening my muscles ... and I would get more out of it since I would have my own individual workout plan. "Everyone reports to the weight room and works on his or her individual goals ... see what I mean?"

Rather than having to change activities when my regular class focused on tasks too difficult for me—like volleyball—I would blend into the situation. There was a catch, however. Kyle continued, "This class isn't normally offered to sophomores, so it's primarily made up of junior and senior boys. You'd be one of only five girls, and the only sophomore. You'd be allowed in the class as an accommodation for your disability."

I stared at Kyle blankly. He knew me well enough to understand that this was indecision mode for me. I didn't shoot the idea down, but I wasn't exactly on his bandwagon, either. "How about if I take you there? You can walk around the class and get a feel for it ... and the kids in it." I gave him a nod in agreement.

The idea of being in a class with mostly boys definitely made me nervous. Kyle and I walked to the weight room, where some twenty-five kids were either working out or standing around. It looked pretty relaxed.

Some athletes might have been taken with the variety of fitness options here. Students could bike, do sit-ups or pull-ups, try the free weights, or walk the treadmill. While I pretended to check out the equipment, I carefully checked out the gender of every student in the room. It was a sea of older boys, none of whom I recognized. Finally, I spotted four girls huddled together by the bench press. As Kyle and I walked near them, they smiled and said, "Hi." *Wow, at least if they're going to check me out, they are nice enough to greet me.*

The idea of being with all of these boys was very intimidating. As Kyle continued to give me the tour, I spotted one boy who looked like he could be Johnny Depp's younger brother. I had never seen him before. *If taking this class means I can see him a few times a week, I'm in!*

71

As Kyle and I left the weight room, he asked, "Well, what do you think?"

"I'll give it a shot."

"That a girl! Really, the weights will make a noticeable difference. This has been on my mind for some time, but I just didn't know … all those boys … But they're great guys. They'll mind their business—do their own thing. This really should improve your walking … "

I smiled. While Kyle rambled on about weight lifting, I thought about how I'd get to watch the Johnny Depp look-alike work out during each phys ed class. Suddenly, I wished I had weight lifting every day.

The next time I saw Kyle, Jennifer, my PT roller-skating instructor, was with him. Jennifer and Kyle informed me that they were going to videotape me walking for some before and after footage. They recorded me walking the length of the gym as well as walking up and down a flight of steps. Of course, my gait was slow—I slouched to the right and seemed bent over as though I was debating if I should pick up a dime off the floor. Climbing the stairway wasn't much different. I held on to the railing the entire time to support myself. *The last thing I need to do is fall, and on camera would make it worse. It'll be hard enough watching this tape, knowing this is the best I can do.*

Over the rest of the school year, I met Kyle three times a week. While he supervised my work on leg extensions, the leg press, the bench press and arm curls, I would sneak glances at the Johnny look-alike. I certainly had spastic muscles, but my hormones were that of a normal teenage girl. Seeing that boy brightened my days.

So while "Johnny" lifted my spirits—made cold walks to the bus stop on phys ed days much easier—I gradually took note: *The weights are really helping me.* I felt like my legs could carry me farther than they had been able to do in the past. I hadn't fallen lately either.

With a couple weeks left in the school year, Jennifer was back with her camcorder to document my improvement. They had me walk the same path as I did a few months prior. When it was all completed, Jennifer smiled and said, "That was really good. You have improved immensely!"

Kyle followed up with, "Say, Jean, would it be okay if I show the before and after footage to another student of mine? She has CP, which is similar to spastic diplegia. And she sure could benefit from weight training if she goes at it like you."

"Sure!" I said enthusiastically. The phys ed change had been a bit overwhelming at first, but I really enjoyed it once I started to feel the benefits. I walked out of the weight room every time much more easily than I walked in. Clearly, all of those strength machines warmed up my muscles and stretched them out in the process. The videotape said it all. The bottom line—I just felt better, and it wasn't merely from the joy of seeing "Johnny" every other day.

Kyle informed me, "If you want to continue the weight training, you can sign up again, in lieu of the regular phys ed classes."

"Really? That would be great." The thought excited me. *I'd really like to keep this up. I feel like I have so much energy—more than I did before. I just wish I could continue this at Blaine High School.*

The boundaries for the school district had changed and next year I would have to attend Anoka High School. I dreaded going back to all those Fred Moore Junior High kids who could be so hurtful. I think I would have done anything to stay at Blaine. For the first time in my life, I felt normal. *I don't have people staring at me because I'm different. If I can stay here at Blaine, I actually think that there is a chance I may have a first date or possibly share a kiss with someone special.* Yes, I admit, these were my educational priorities. There were a few boys at Blaine who actually paid attention to me and possibly found me attractive, despite my abnormalities.

The most challenging part of my school day had always been the walk home from the bus stop. As the day progressed, my walking got worse. I slumped forward, both knees turned inward and my left arm tightened up—the chicken wing. To add to the burden of finding my way home after an exhausting day, I had to carry my school bag. It weighed just a pound or two, but it felt like a trunk load of groceries. I already dreaded getting off the bus in front of those old junior high classmates. In my mind, they were eternally immature, and lacked the empathy to consider that life for me was just a little harder—at least physically.

As I did in junior high, I left my Blaine classes five minutes early. With the hallways to myself, I found my way to my locker and retrieved my jacket, which was always difficult to put on. As I put my right arm into the sleeve I almost always lost my balance, staggering back and forth in something that looked like a two-year-old's "potty dance."

The crisp air always recharged me after a cooped-up day of school. I exited the building and the intense sun blinded me as I walked the half block to the curb where all the buses were parked. Catching the evening ride was so easy during my first year of high school because prompt St. Nick parked in the same spot each and every afternoon. Throughout my years prior to Blaine, getting home was not so predictable. As I frantically left Fred Moore Junior High, I had to search the bright yellow convoy of twenty-five buses—my driver seemed to be hiding his vehicle in a different spot every day. Occasionally, I'd luck out and find my bus driver parked first in line. But more often than not, I'd stumble almost the full two blocks before catching my balance to climb those three tricky steps to a crowded mass of preteens who had no problem announcing, "You can't sit here—this is saved for ___ (anyone but me)."

On St. Nick's bus, I generally sat by myself and read a paperback book. I'd chat with the other sophomores for the first fifteen minutes of the ride, but as they slowly dispersed, I'd retreat to my book for the remaining thirty minutes. I spent about two hours a day on that bus—first one on in the morning and dead last in the evening. Thanks to St. Nick and some nice classmates, it was a stress-free ride.

This bus driver was so sensitive to my physical limitations. By the second week of school, he attempted to navigate our dead-end cul-de-sac.

"Say, sit a little longer ... I'll getcha to your driveway."

This was no easy feat. The narrow design of the cul-de-sac prevented even a Y-turn. My driver couldn't quite turn around, so he eventually backed the bus up to get off my street. His intentions were wonderful. *Well, he tried. Nice to be dropped off a few steps from my front door, but I better not get used to this.*

The next afternoon, St. Nick surprised me when I stood to exit the bus at the end of my street.

"Hey, sit back down for one more minute. I've got another idea."

I observed while he maneuvered that rigid, oversized yellow box backwards down Martin Court. He broke my watchful gaze when he suddenly opened the door.

"There you go, young lady!"

This was my cue to stand up. I slowly descended the steep three steps, then paused and turned just before he closed the door.

"Thank you," I said, smiling.

"Anytime," he replied.

I know he doesn't have to do this. He's probably risking his job. No bus driver had ever taken the time for such an act of kindness for me or anyone else, for that matter. He did this every day for the rest of the year, and no matter what kind of day I was having, I made sure I thanked him. And before drifting off to sleep, I thanked God for making Santa Claus my bus driver.

* * *

Well, St. Nick's service is over—this is going to stink!

I was thoroughly pissed off for my official first day at Anoka High School. Anger churned in my stomach as I climbed an unfamiliar bus entrance to face the inevitable transfer to another school. The boundary change I prayed for all summer never occurred, so I had no choice but to bounce back into the student body that triggered only miserable memories for me. *God, please give me the strength to get through this unwanted change. Help me to see the good in others and help others to see that I'm just a normal teenager like them. More than anything, please guide my words, because there's a good chance that I'm going to say something that I may regret from being so angry with this boundary change.*

As my bus took its final turn into the parking lot, my fury festered. I was ready to hit something, or someone, if I heard one mocking remark. I'm sure I had a scowl on my face—one for which my parents would have surely scolded me. The only consolation with this change was that my best friend, Amy, had to endure the transfer as well. I sat sulking on the bus, fantasizing a sudden turn into

Blaine High School. Amy took a parallel ride, dreaming of a detour to Coon Rapids Senior High. Despite the fact that we had been in different schools, we both loved our sophomore years, and resented the abrupt switch. *Misery loves company—at least Amy will complain with me.*

Sharon and Stockamp—consolation number two: Our last names put our lockers in the same locker bay. Frankly, I was relieved to find Amy so quickly in the mass of Anoka students. After a greeting of gratitude for having each other, we protested our displacement, "What are we doing here? This is so unfair!"

A jolt of joy hit when we realized we were assigned the same lunch period, but angst for completely different class schedules fueled my bad attitude. Amy's presence in this building was about the only motivation I had to return the next day.

Alone, I set out to find my first classroom. The familiar sound of boys laughing broke my focus. I hesitated, and risked a sidelong glance at a group of teenagers huddled together near some lockers. Sure enough, one of them was imitating my gait. He dragged one leg and hit his arm against his chest. *My chicken wing, already? Did I look like that so early in the day?* I pretended to not notice. *I'm not going to let these clowns get me down ... but honestly how can't I? I'm human. I have feelings. Just because I'm disabled doesn't mean that I don't get sad. Lord, I don't think I can go through this again. Please, make them stop.*

My mind raced with anger toward students who believed they had a license to ridicule anyone they deemed inferior. What made them think that a physical disability meant my feelings were null and void? Did they believe my heart was detached—surgically removed, like the leg muscles cut years ago at the hospital? I wanted to turn and yell something, but what good would it do? So, I practiced in my mind for the hundredth time ...

Can't you see the damage you do? Can't you tell that a small piece of me is bruised every time you mimic me? You slam me ... like I'm not even human to you ... I'm here for your enjoyment ... go ahead, make fun, enjoy at my expense. You aren't physically harming me or even saying mean things to my face. So, if it's behind my back, it's okay, right? No harm done?

Their simple act of imitating my walk brought instant attention to the obvious—that I am different ... that I will always be different ... that their jokes drew a line all around me ... that some people would never be comfortable crossing that line to seek my friendship ... that I may not ever have a boyfriend, or get married, or have children ...

Day one of this school year and I had already confronted all these heavy thoughts. *Can I possibly ignore them for 169 more days?* I sensed this year would be the ultimate test of my self-control and my faith in God.

* * *

Now that I was sixteen years old, Mom said that I needed to learn how to drive. Without St. Nick as my bus driver, I welcomed the idea of taking the car to school. However, once seated behind the wheel of Mom's car, apprehension hijacked me. The notion of relying on my impaired arms and legs to command a vehicle along Minnesota's busy highways—quite honestly, I was petrified.

At my last neurology appointment with Dr. Anderson, Mom had asked if I would be able to drive. He hesitated, then stated, "Well, put her in the car and have her try it. If it goes well, she can. If she can't, she can't." *Hmm ... profound, Doctor. But what if I realize I can't drive while I'm behind the wheel? Will you be available to patch me up after the accident?!*

Dad drove us home from that appointment, and I sensed everyone's disappointment from Dr. Anderson's response. Clearly, Mom and Dad wanted a simple "yes" or "no" too.

My grandma was the first to accept Dr. Anderson's wishy-washy advice. She offered to take me behind the wheel. "Let's try the church parking lot, Jeanie." This sounded a lot better than starting with Mom or Dad as my driving instructor. Grandma would be more relaxed, and would definitely make me laugh if I goofed up. Plus, how much damage could I do in a church parking lot? God would surely watch over us there!

One Saturday morning, Grandma drove me to the church parking lot as promised. She parked the car and we both got out. We walked around the front of the black Ford Taurus, trading positions—I buckled up behind the wheel, and Grandma snapped into the front passenger seat.

"Okay, Jeannie. Remember, your right foot should rest on the brake. You're going to start the car, put it in gear, then slowly move your foot to the gas pedal."

I patiently listened, even though I had watched Mom and Dad drive my entire life. Since it was Grandma, I didn't give her any attitude, despite the fact that these basics had been drilled into my head in driver's ed.

"Now, start slowly. We've got all morning. There's no reason to hurry," Grandma advised.

I was fine with this. *The parking lot's a perfect driving course.* I had to dodge one parked car and several light posts. But there were no people that I could injure—other than the two of us. It was a crystal clear day with green leaves in full bloom on the churchyard trees. I put my foot on the brake, turned the key, and gradually took the car out of park.

"Okay, Jeanie, you can take your foot off the brake."

Grandma's voice guided me as I cautiously followed her soothing commands. I was driving! I crawled around St. Pat's parking lot, which transformed into a concrete roadway made especially for me. I noticed every crack and curve—every patch of pothole created by Minnesota weather. How could this parking lot, which I pulled into every Sunday morning and Wednesday night for years, suddenly look so different? After a half an hour of driving around in circles, Grandma informed me that it was time to move on to a bigger challenge.

"The road?" I ask her with trepidation.

"No," she replied, with equal concern in her voice. "The cemetery."

Smiling, she added, "You can't kill anyone there."

We both laughed as I steered our Taurus into the cemetery, located on a patch of property adjacent to the church parking lot. I cruised around the oval track several times without incident. After a few laps, we decided this was enough for one day. "It's probably best if I drive us back home," Grandma suggested. "You need something for your next lesson, right?"

Once Grandma initiated me into the world of driving, my mom took over from there. Every Saturday morning, mother and daughter headed to St. Patrick's Church, but suddenly I was the chauffeur on the way there, as well.

"There's very little traffic going in that direction," Mom noticed—something we both liked. Grandma had helped me overcome the initial anxiety of driving. But I still feared being alone at the wheel. Mom gave me the practice I needed to believe that this was a skill I could conquer.

Like making a varsity sports team, or performing with a dance-line group, I had placed driving on that mental list of "not in my lifetime." I entered plenty of items on my "must accomplish" list—like going to college and keeping good grades. And despite my rough start at Anoka High School, I remained optimistic with my mental list of "maybe—don't give up quite yet," which included having a prom date or a steady boyfriend. But driving … this was something I never considered—a task blocked from my paradigm of possibilities.

As I drove one morning down Hanson Boulevard toward church, my mom advised me, "Take it slow. We're in no hurry."

I was traveling about five miles under the speed limit, which didn't bother me, until I caught the car in my rearview mirror. "Mom, there's someone behind me."

"You just worry about you," she reminded me. "Stay in your lane," which I must add, was stated to me at least one thousand times while I learned to drive. (I never did leave my lane, my entire first year of driving.)

I slowly approached the oncoming stop sign.

"Mom, what's that car doing?"

Despite the fact that this was a single-lane stretch of roadway, the car that had been tailgating me pulled up to my mom's window. A big lady with long, greasy black hair rolled down her window and yelled, "Learn how to drive," then sped ahead through the intersecting street.

My mom, who remains cool in the most difficult situations, and who rarely showed anger through most of my childhood, was clearly annoyed by this woman.

"If she wasn't so big and didn't look so mean, I would have yelled at her," she stated with a scowl rarely shown to anyone.

"What would you have said?" I asked.

"Wash your hair!" We both burst out laughing as I made my turn into the familiar church parking lot.

* * *

I passed! I passed! I silently celebrated as I left the DMV one summer morning in 1993. *I am a legal Minnesota driver! Thank you, God! I never thought this would happen.*

I pulled into the parking space with the testing officer that day, and she turned to me and stated, "You are a very good driver."

"Thanks!" I replied, not only pleased, but reassured.

After the test, my parents gave me the keys to Mom's car and told me to drive to Amy's house. I pulled into her driveway and she looked so surprised. "Who brought you?"

"I drove myself."

"What? You took your test today without telling me?!" I had a feeling Amy would be hurt that I had not shared my appointment date.

I explained how I didn't know I would be taking my driver's exam that day.

"I didn't want Mom to tell me when it would be." I could see that I was only adding to Amy's confusion.

"I knew that I would be so nervous. You know how I can't sleep when I'm nervous … which causes spasticity and tremors … which makes my control even worse … yada, yada."

The light bulb went on as Amy listened.

"Jeez, the things you have to think about … I can't imagine not knowing when my driver's test is gonna be … having my mom spring it on me like that."

"I don't know ... life's just easier when I get enough sleep."

I knew I couldn't take this test any other way. Mom woke me at 7:00 A.M. and told me to get dressed for my exam. My mom understood me like no one else could or ever would. She knew that sleep was a necessity or my muscles would fight every move. She also knew just how to push me ... how to get me to accomplish things I didn't believe were possible. Dad was good at this too. But Mom had driven with me so much she had a master plan to get me through that test—and it worked!

Despite my test success, and the complimentary feedback from the DMV, I dreaded the drive alone to Amy's house, or anywhere. If Mom was in the car, I gladly took the keys. Until one morning, my dad pushed the issue and offered me Mom's car for school.

"No, thanks. I'll take the bus."

My dad turned to me, "Jean, here are the keys to Mom's car. You're driving to school from now on. You don't need to take the bus."

"But I don't want to drive to school," I snapped.

My dad looked at me with sternness in his eyes and I knew this was not a battle that I could win.

"Other kids would give anything to have a car to drive to school and not take the bus." I knew he was right. I wasn't ungrateful—just chicken.

I took the keys and drove to school, arriving more than thirty minutes early to avoid morning traffic. I parked the car in the closest handicap space. My walking wasn't too bad in the morning, but by the end of the day, I would be slow and mechanical. Making my way across campus to my parked car without drawing a ton of attention would become my daily goal. As I passed my bumper, I laughed at the "Blaine Football" sticker. *That won't go over well—better tell the office I parked here.*

By the end of the day, I fought to get my coat on—more than usual. I grabbed my notebook and car keys from my locker, and struggled every step of the way to the car. I frequently felt the decline in my legs, but this afternoon was particularly memorable. I was bent over more than usual and my left hamstring and calf muscle were exceptionally tight. As I stepped over the curb near the car, I caught my right toe on the concrete, and fell to my knees. I slowly got to my feet, glancing around to see if anyone saw my stumble. Jason Cooke and a girl whose name I don't remember approached me.

"Do you need help?" he asked. He was one of those kind kids from way back at Crooked Lake Elementary. I knew I was safe. None of the kids I knew in elementary school ever made fun of me. We must have created a bond that I just couldn't seem to get with new students.

"No, thanks. I'll be okay," I said, noticing my jeans were wet at the knees from the melted snow. I was not one to accept help—this hadn't changed from elementary school. My reply to deny assistance, from even a trusted classmate like Jason, was almost an instinct—a knee-jerk reaction whenever someone offered a hand in kindness. Independence, or the illusion of it, trumped any desire I had to accept even a gesture toward simplifying my struggle. Perhaps I refused to feel any more powerless than I was. Sometimes I believed this was all I had over the others—my strong will to overcome the physical workout that accompanied an uncooperative body.

So, once again I said, "No—I'm fine … but thanks." *Earn their respect … then, always an attitude of gratitude for not kicking me when I'm down.*

Jason handed me my notebook and I reached into my pocket for Mom's keys. *I'm only a few steps away. I can do this.*

The three of us parted ways as I unlocked my car. Fighting my balance, I opened the door, but my right leg seemed glued to the ground. I lifted and pushed it into the front seat, as the rest of my body fell sideways into the car. I used the steering wheel for leverage, and shimmied my hips to a sitting position. *Shut the door,* I thought, and I released a sigh so sad sounding, I wanted to cry. *Lord, please keep me strong. I want to cry, but if I start, I won't stop … and then I won't be able to see the road … and then I'll be stuck here even longer. Suck it up, and start the car.*

Just then, someone tapped on my window. I looked up from the ignition to see a parent—no one I knew personally, but clearly the mom of someone from Anoka High School. I rolled down my window. *I'm sure she saw me fall and wants to make sure I'm all right.*

"Should you be driving?" she stated bluntly, her big blonde curls blowing in the wind.

"Yes, I'm fine," I answered quickly, although this was not the question I had anticipated.

"I don't think you should be driving. Give me your keys," she said, holding out her left hand.

"I said that I'm fine." I frowned in anger as I read her mind. *She thinks I'm drunk.*

She backed up a little as my power window began to close. She finally stepped away from my car, and moved in the direction of the school's front door. Once even with the hood of my mom's car, she glanced in the direction of the handicap sign, and stopped dead in her tracks. As I put the car in reverse, her head dropped toward the ground. She turned to face me again, but this time with an apologetic smile.

I can hear the voice in *her* head now—*That student isn't drunk. She's disabled. I feel like a fool.*

But my own little voice retaliated quickly. *Yes, you should feel bad.* This incident—an act of concern on her part, a responsible gesture if the student was indeed drunk—was the worst experience of my life to date. In her sudden judgment as I stumbled into the car, I gained an insight that I had clearly ignored ... I was defined and judged completely by my disability. I confronted the knowledge that I could not fake my way through spastic diplegia. If I ever entertained the delusion that people didn't notice, that on a good day, I could cover, it was gone now. I lost that dream in a brief encounter at Anoka's high school parking lot.

I backed up the car, abruptly shifted into drive, and let my tears fall down my face. *Really, God. Is this what I have to deal with? Does everyone see me like such a freak? Why did you make me like this? Why me?* I had waited to leave until the parking lot was empty—thankfully, no one could see me cry. *I don't have to be strong. I don't care if the road is blurry.* Instinct drove me home that afternoon, and in true Jeanie fashion, I stopped crying just as I entered my driveway. I set the keys on the front table, climbed the stairs to my room, and shut the door.

Agoraphobia at the Podium

Junior year at Anoka High School provided plenty of challenges, but one in particular caused me more trauma than some chicken-wing imitation by a locker-bay bully. Junior year at Anoka required every student to pass a presentation test that would separate the true egos from the frauds. Although I didn't identify with either end of this spectrum, I feared that my shallow confidence would fail me just when I needed some real self-esteem.

Every English 11 student had to research a topic of his/her choice, and then give a formal speech to the class regarding the findings. From Day 1 of the school year, I maintained a delusion of denial. I managed to block the image of me all alone in front of the room … my shaky grasp trying to steady a three-by-five note card … my phony facial expression and intermittent eye contact having no impact on a room full of patronizing peers … my speech day was pure fantasy. Why think about something more than half the year away?

But the second semester had arrived.

The teacher won't make me do it … I'll be sick on the day I'm scheduled to speak … I'll wait until word of the redistricting goes through and I'll get transferred back to Blaine …

Yet, as the months were torn from the classroom calendar, my greatest fear was becoming a reality.

I was tempted to talk with the guidance counselor—I could claim that my condition affected my speech. *Students won't be able to understand me … I slur when I'm nervous.* Although I told a great lie in my head, I could never use my diagnosis as an excuse to dodge what others were required to do. *Spastic diplegia would not excuse me from this graduation requirement, so I might as well get it over with.*

Yet, every time I thought about getting in front of my class, I sensed my muscles tensing up. *How will I possibly stand at the front of the room with thirty kids watching me? Lord, I need you more now than ever before.* For all the months I deterred and dreaded the assignment, I was now thinking and planning it every moment of every day. I just wanted the thing behind me!

Halfway through the quarter, my English 11 teacher finally instructed us on the steps for the research projects. We all began searching a topic and prepping our findings for our five- to seven-minute speech. I wavered between basic anger ... *I just don't understand why this speech is necessary! I'm doing the research and writing the paper—why isn't that enough!* ... and self-reprimand for being such a coward. *Why am I so nervous to do this? I love talking to people. I talk way too much in this class. What's the big deal?* But ever since that day I read my short story to the fourth-grade class, I had a fear of speaking in front of groups.

My fourth-grade teacher had us complete a one-page creative writing assignment about, of all things, a fox. Our teacher read each story to the students, and then asked them to vote for their favorite. This charged my competitive side—I enjoyed writing, so I wanted desperately to win. I put my heart into the fox story, and sure enough, my piece was selected by my peers. I think it meant even more to me because the teacher had left each piece anonymous. I was elated and proud!

Upon winning the contest, my teacher reminded me that I would be reading my piece to each class in my grade. At that age, I still enjoyed show-and-tell, so the concept of reading in front of these classrooms excited me.

I rotated from room to room, sharing my tale, and getting high praise and loud applause from three consecutive fourth-grade groups! I stood tall at the front of each room and shared my story in a loud, clear voice. I was eager to share my final reading with

Mr. Key's class—my best friend Stephanie was in that section. She would share in my joy ... I hoped I had saved my best performance for last.

I entered Stephanie's classroom, and began reading my story. About halfway through, I looked up and saw my friend looking back at me with a genuine smile. As though someone had flipped a switch, I suddenly felt my presence at the front of this room ... I became cognizant for the first time of a room full of kids with all eyes on me as I read. My hands began to shake ... my eyes could not read the print on the notebook paper ... I stuttered and paused at inappropriate times. I didn't know if I could go on.

I stopped, turned, and with pleading eyes, looked at the teacher standing next to me, and tried to convey, "Please, let me stop."

The teacher smiled down at me, nodded and said, "Go on ... "

I glanced again at Stephanie, noticed her concerned look, and with my shaky voice and trembling paper, I finished my story ... something I suddenly wished I had never written.

Although my fourth-grade creative writing experience had ended on a foul note, I had long forgotten the embarrassment of fumbling my way through that story in front of Stephanie and others. Of course, it all came racing back to me as I visualized my junior English presentation. The disastrous conclusion to that fourth-grade production became a vivid example to me—*I am* NOT *a public speaker!* I didn't bother to recall the three almost flawless rounds of storytelling that had occurred prior to entering Stephanie's classroom. I was convinced that speeches were for actors and divas ... not for cowards like me. *I'm just no good at this stuff ... I spend my days trying to blend in—not stand out as a disabled student. My shaky hands will draw every ounce of focus to my disability. It doesn't matter what I talk about—kids won't hear a word I say.* Convinced they would all simply stare at me, I imagined their concerned looks ... wondering if my weak legs would hold me up for five minutes. *I just have to get this over with—I need to go first, and have my last speech behind me forever.*

For the next month, I put my heart and soul into researching agoraphobia. Mike helped me pick the topic.

"It'll be interesting. People don't know much about it, but there have been a lot of studies done. Some really famous people had this phobia." Mike had been paying attention in some college class, I guess.

When he first mentioned it to me, I had never heard of the word, much less knew what it meant. But when I looked it up and learned it was a term for those who are fearful of leaving the protection of their homes, I was intrigued. As someone who popped up before the alarm sounded, and had trudged through the January wind to get to the bus stop, I could hardly relate to those who hid from life's challenges. I rarely felt the desire to sleep in, or feared the unknown potential of a new day. Even while confronting the fear of this speech assignment, I still had that natural curiosity that drew me into my schoolwork. I couldn't imagine a fear so strong that it would handicap a competent person.

Mike was right—this was odd, but many would either empathize, or, like me, wonder how such anxiety could cripple someone. I started my study and found many famous and talented people—from Emily Dickinson to Woody Allen to Sigmund Freud himself—had fought this debilitating condition.

Precisely, agoraphobia is "extreme or irrational fear of a situation where escape may be difficult; it is characterized by panic, and avoidance of wide open spaces or crowded public places." *I may not want to talk about it, but I know that the research will be a big portion of my grade. I'll hate speech day, but I know I can write a darn good paper.*

I was petrified to stand in front of my peers for five minutes and talk while they daydreamed. Yet, deep down inside, I knew I was being silly. *For heaven's sake, anyone can talk for five minutes. Get over it!* But the more I scolded myself, the more my confidence went down. I'd visualize Mr. Evan calling out my name—"Jean Sharon ... you're up." I would feel my nerves taking over. I would walk from my desk to the front of the room, slower than any student should. I would hold my note cards—a crutch without which I'd fail for sure—and shake uncontrollably while the few audience members polite enough to listen flashed condescending smiles of discomfort, thinking, "Come on, Jean, you can do this."

I would think about the other kids who might be dreading this … maybe I wasn't alone in my fear. *It's one thing to be nervous and get a dry mouth, or have your voice quiver a bit. It's a whole different thing when your entire body shakes.* I just couldn't pep-talk myself into this.

"Remember, you can't use the podium! No hiding from us." Mr. Evan reminded us of this condition just days before we presented. I'm sure this mandate was communicated when the assignment was first outlined to us, but how could I remember all the particulars when I was scared to death? *Why would he do this? Can't he see that a podium would shield and protect me from a total spaz attack?*

One week prior to my scheduled presentation, I began to practice giving my speech to my mom every night. She said that the more I practiced, the less nervous I would be. I understood what she was saying, but practice seemed to heighten my nervousness. *I hate thinking about this every single day in class, and now after school too. Enough with the practice—I just want it over with!*

"Remember, you can use note cards—just don't be too dependent on them." Mr. Evan had no idea that this was a useless tool for me. *Once I start shaking, I won't be able to read what's on the cards. Plus, there's a really good chance that my arms will tighten up so much that I won't be able to rotate the cards from front to back. I suppose I could just write on the front sides … but what if I drop them? I can't even go there.*

The day before my presentation, I was feeling pretty good about my speech. Mom was right, of course—the practice made my factual recall easier. My confidence was high—*it's a really good speech! I know it by heart and can give it effectively, at least to my mom. When the teacher walks into class, I'm going to ask if I can go today! Why wait … I'm not nervous, and he might want to get things underway!*

Mr. Evan walked in and I instantly lost my confidence. I kept my mouth shut, and for the next fifty minutes, I listened to him teach the same stuff we had been hearing all quarter. He gave us even more presentation pointers and informed the class that he was looking forward to listening to us over the next three days. I wasn't sure what I was going to do—*agoraphobia may hit me with a vengeance tomorrow morning!* Yet skipping my speech was not a choice.

* * *

All of this seems quite ironic now—now that I have a communications degree from Winona State University, and have learned to channel my anxiety over public speaking into positive and controlled energy. I know it seems absurd, an utter lie perhaps, when I say I actually chose organizational communications as my major. It sounded strange when I first discovered that the major even existed. No one can say we don't learn from our failures.

An F?! I'll have to transfer schools or change my major.

In fact, I was on my second major by this time my sophomore year.

The paralegal field was why I came to Winona State University in the first place. But after changing my major once already, I reminisced about my decision to come here. While many classmates chose a college for no other reason than it was popular with high school friends, I had chosen to go it alone. I picked WSU, and then learned that some great girls from my class were indeed going there too. I moved into my dorm, settled into campus life, and despite a struggle with pinning down my major, I was not about to transfer elsewhere just because I failed one required course.

I can't get around the professor who gave me the F ... he's the only guy who teaches that class. I probably should not be majoring in something that is such a struggle anyway. I grabbed a copy of the WSU course catalogue of majors. Well, here goes. I'm leaving it in God's hands. Whatever I open up to will be my new major. Not exactly a scientific method for choosing a career, but I was ready to leave it to fate ... or should I say *faith*. Drumroll ... I opened the big book of majors to ... art.

What?! I can't major in art! For obvious reasons, my motor skills would prevent me from taking art as a serious study. I hated art classes as a kid, only because they were so hard for me. I closed the big book and tried again.

Don't fail me now, God. Drumroll ... this time, the big pages parted and I paused long enough to consider "mass communications" on the left page and "organizational communications" on the right. *I didn't know that WSU had these two majors.* As I read the descriptions and requirements for each of these fields, I sensed some hope. I had already taken many of the classes listed due to my previous majors, paralegal and public relations. *Well ... at least there's some overlap. Maybe this will work out after all.* But my hope was quickly countered with fear as I spotted "Intro to Speech" and "Public Speaking" on the lists of requirements for both of these communications majors. This was logical, of course ... but these classes provided a huge hurdle—one that I didn't think I had the legs to jump.

I held the white catalog opened to the Cs while I contemplated closing it for one more round of Course Catalogue Roulette. *I could keep doing this until I find a career that I like.* But I decided to leave it in God's hands. Not that I would blame God if I threw up during my first speech ... but I felt compelled to trust His guidance. I registered for my next semester classes, and "Intro to Speech" topped my list.

Eventually, I would graduate with no minor since this degree essentially combined mass communications, human resources, and public relations into one package deal. However, on the eve of my agoraphobia speech, with Emily Dickinson-like symptoms so pronounced that I considered crawling under my bed for the next decade, I would have chosen to drink hemlock, like Socrates, before I would have ever agreed to a speech-related college major. All of this high school hoopla was in fact leading to a communications degree ... proof of life's unpredictable nature. But, of course, who would have believed that I would one day live without spastic diplegia?

* * *

Speech Day, Grade 11, had arrived! I told the students sitting next to me that I was incredibly nervous.

"What? You'll do fine," one of them spouted back.

"No, actually, I shake really bad when I'm nervous—like, worse than usual. If I fall over, don't laugh, okay?" I thought they would laugh this off, but surprisingly, most had rather serious looks on their faces.

"I just wish I could use a podium."

This was Kevin's cue. I could tell this was enough for him to want to do something to help me.

Kevin, it is worth adding, was super cute. He looked at me with his green eyes and stated, "I'll ask the teacher if you can use a podium. What's the big deal?"

Before I could protest, he was out in the hallway, talking to our teacher, clearly requesting the podium for me … explaining that I had "special circumstances" that should be accommodated.

Who is this guy? I hardly know him, yet he'll ask for something extra to help me when I don't have the guts to ask myself?

Kevin returned to the classroom with the teacher just as efficiently as he had left, and within a moment, a portable podium was in his hands. He placed the podium on the table in the front of the room—my cue to get ready.

As Kevin returned to his desk, he informed me that "the podium won't keep you from falling, but it will help you if you place your hands on top of it."

Swirling words from my speech were floating around in my head, along with other spontaneous thoughts that might impede my presentation. *I always thought Kevin was cute, but I never thought that he could be so thoughtful. It amazes me—some kids are so incredibly nice to me. How would I know this unless I needed them for some reason? People like Kevin make up for the mean kids.*

Mr. Evan made it clear that class was starting.

"It's our first day of speeches … " he rambled on with some introductory stuff, but I was still trying to fathom Kevin's kindness. I suddenly see Julian, another student I rarely talk to, smile at me. His smile was genuine. *He can tell that I am nervous … he seems to know that I might vomit or pee in my pants.* His smile was enough … he gave me another boost needed to start the speech.

"Jean Sharon—you're on." My teacher's clipboard listed me at the top of the chart.

I walked to the front of the room, turned, and faced my classmates. Before the silence could get to me, I started in with a line I must have delivered to my mom a hundred times …

"Imagine yourself afraid to leave the safety and security of your own home … "

I don't recall much more of the speech—just that first line. Yes, there were nerves. Yes, there was shaking. But I did it ... I spoke fluently, and without a lapse of memory, or a crisis of confidence.

The class clapped as I walked back to my desk. I didn't fall. I didn't vomit or wet myself. All in all, I'd call it a success.

I sat back in my desk, satisfied that no one had to call 911. Students around me turned and told me I did a great job. They were all supporting me, just as they would a good friend. This felt nice—not just to be done, but to draw those reactions from others. Whether or not what they said was true—although my intuition told me I did fine—no one had cracked a joke. No one had laughed at me. *Was I bringing out some good in them because I was vulnerable and needed their support?* I truly believe this was the first time that I had ever acknowledged such a question ... that a speech could somehow be more significant to the listeners because of the presenter's unusual circumstances. I didn't mull on that insight for too long, because it was now my turn to listen ... and I would do this with the mutual respect and kindness they gave me.

Scoot on Down to Winona

My junior year of high school became *The Year of Projects*. After conquering the dreaded speech in English class, my next mission was to explore life after high school. Of course, for me, this meant researching college choices. I always knew that I would go away to school. It was just a matter of where I would go and what I should study. I didn't take long to trim down my options to Winona State University in Winona, Minnesota, since I wanted a paralegal degree. This program wasn't offered at every state college, so Winona won the honor of my application by default. Once my research and decision had been made, I secured an appointment for the second part of the project—a career planning session with my guidance counselor. Although I felt prepared when I went to see her, I had not anticipated her reaction to my plans.

Ms. Thomas was less than thrilled with my decision to move away from home. She strongly suggested that I stay home and attend the local community college. "I don't think you'll be able to make it away at school. It's a big move for anyone to live in a dorm and adjust to campus living away from their parents. Talk with your folks about the community college option. I'm sure they'll agree."

I left school that afternoon feeling stunned and defeated. I sat at the oak kitchen table while Mom made dinner as tears rolled down my cheeks. My mom turned to face me just as Mike came down the stairs and entered the kitchen. They both gave me a sympathetic look as they quickly glanced at one another trying to figure out what the problem was.

"I'm not going to college," I announced.

Mike, who had just finished college, and had recently moved home while he settled into a new job, asked, "Why not?"

"I'll never be able to do it," I said as my mom continued cooking.

"If you want to go to college, you can do it," Mike interrupted. "And if you don't want to go to college, no one is saying that you have to." I could tell by my mom's expression that Mike was reading her mind and speaking for both of them.

"I want to become a paralegal. Winona State's got the only program, but Ms. Thomas said that there is no way I will make it away from home."

Mike assured me that if I put my mind to it, I would manage just fine at college. "There are so many students in wheelchairs at school with way more problems than you. Don't let that stop you." He continued to share with me that his guidance counselor had told him he would never get through college either … "and I made it." Then he added, "Tom was told by his counselor that he'd never be more than an auto mechanic. Don't listen to her. Do what you want to do."

I don't recall being overly excited or pumped up at the end of that conversation. But looking back, I'm glad that Mike spoke so assertively to me. I knew that at least my family supported my decision, and although I had doubts and fears, I knew that God would be by my side during this entire journey. I wasn't going to let someone stop me from fulfilling, or at least attempting to fulfill, my dreams. Besides, I couldn't live with Mom and Dad forever.

During the winter of my senior year of high school, my parents took me on several college tours. Just as my research indicated, Winona State had the only paralegal program. However, I wanted to keep my options open. Maybe there was a better career path for me than what Winona State had to offer. My parents and Mike thought that I should take a closer look at Southwest State in Marshall, Minnesota (Mike's college), since it catered to students with disabilities, especially those in wheelchairs. I frowned on this option—*Marshall's in the middle of nowhere.* Yet, I agreed to a tour since deep down I knew this school would be the easiest for me to navigate.

Before we toured each campus, Mom would make an appointment with the school's mobility advisor. Southwest State was no different. We met with this advisor in a small, dark office in the lower level of an old building. It felt like a scene out of a mob movie. As we took the gloomy and aged stairwell down, I imagined meeting a gangster who broke people's legs, not helped those who couldn't use theirs.

The massive mafia man sat on one side of the table—my parents and I slid into the chairs directly across from him. My mom started in with a summary of all the accommodations I currently received at Anoka High School: extra time between classes, an extra set of books stored at home … He interrupted, then kindly clarified why these accommodations became obsolete in a college setting, "Extra time between classes won't be necessary. Most students don't take back-to-back classes."

My mom went on to explain that I have difficulty walking in the afternoon and evening and that carrying heavy books wasn't realistic.

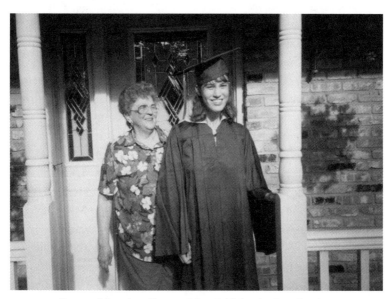

Jean and Grandma Sharon at Jean's high school graduation

"Is there a possibility of having students help Jean? Like student volunteers—to carry her books across campus to class?" He listened carefully to my mom's concerns, paused, and then explained her worries away once again.

"We don't have any services like that here." He went on to tell us that this would be a time for me to gain more independence. "You're going to need a scooter," he stated directly at me.

This was not a question. This was a statement. A man who had only known me for ten minutes was telling me to give up on my legs—something I'd been fighting to save my whole life. I could feel my parents experiencing the same emotional response as me.

"She doesn't need a scooter," my dad affirmed. "She just needs some help getting to classes."

"I understand what you're saying," the mobility counselor said, leaning back slightly. "There are a handful of students at Southwest State who already use scooters. You'll see, Jean. This will allow you to go where you want, when you want."

We were informed that the scooter was not optional if I intended to enroll in this college. I felt anger taking over my ability to listen and refute this man's ultimatum. Then sadness stifled my anger as we thanked the counselor for his time and started our ride back to Andover.

I had miles to think about all the questions this campus visit raised about my college future … and more. *I want to go away to college, but is it possible? Am I being realistic? Ms. Thomas thinks I need to go to the community college. Now I have this advisor telling me I can only go to Southwest State if I give in to a scooter. I don't want a scooter. I don't want to stick out like a disabled student, and a scooter will guarantee that. Why can't I just have someone help me carry my books? Why does this have to be so complicated? Why can't I be normal? Other kids go off to college and they don't have to worry about how they will get to class, or how they will carry their books. Why do I have to be any different? God, please guide me in finding these answers. Please, tell me what to do!*

My parents gave me a few quiet miles for my own thoughts, but then interrupted so we could talk over the scooter question.

"Maybe it's not such a bad idea, Jean, no matter where you end up going," my dad spoke up. "It'll allow you to get around campus on your own. No matter how late it is in the evening, or how badly your walking gets on a given day, you won't feel stranded if you have a scooter to get you home quickly."

But I don't want a scooter!!! I heard myself shouting, but it was only my internal voice.

I'm sure the silent car ride told my parents that there was hope I would once again comply.

* * *

About a month before I left for Winona State, my first and ultimately final college choice, Dad arrived home from work with a scooter. I couldn't help but feel sadness at the sight of it.

Tom seemed to come out of nowhere to jump on board for the scooter's first spin. He rode up and down the driveway, turning circles with a big smile on his face, bragging about its horsepower, and claiming it would pass even the seniors on campus.

"Try it!" he cheered as he hopped off. "You can run over any freshman who gets in your way."

I sat on the scooter, spied the two levers—forward and backward gears—then noticed the turtle and rabbit symbols that indicated the speed. *What the heck … this looks like a kid's toy.*

"What are you looking at … it's easy to drive. Get going," Tom encouraged me.

I started out slowly, but gradually sped up, and rode around the driveway, like Tom had. *I can go faster than he did.* I hit the reverse lever, then quickly pushed the button to go forward causing the vehicle to pop a wheelie. Tom and I doubled over in laughter. He knew if I could make a joke of this, all would be okay.

* * *

I can feel the butterflies in my stomach. Lonnie had a firm grip on the wheel of her car as we drove away from Anoka, our high school years in the rearview mirror. Neither one of us noticed the towering bluffs along Highway 61, positioned as fortress walls over the sailboats on Lake Pepin. We were too focused on keeping up with my parents as both cars followed the winding Mississippi River road south toward Winona. Our lives were about to change forever, and both of us seemed intent on our vision of dorm life, rather than the sights we left behind.

"Okay, Lonnie, it's just the two of us until Angie gets here in a week. Best part—no parents, no brothers. Just us, and a bunch of college kids. This is going to be awesome!" I was pumped for the change, and covering anxiety with my best bravado.

A green Minnesota state sign informed us that the city of Winona was thirty miles away. We turned to face each other, and squealed in chorus, "We're almost there!"

I couldn't have been happier or more relieved to be sharing this experience with Lonnie Swanson. I had been friends with her since the day I came home from the hospital nursery, eighteen years ago. She lived across the dirt road from our house on Vintage Street. And although we moved a few miles away when I was three, and attended a different elementary school, our friendship grew stronger every year.

A couple of signs—Reduced Speed Limit and Winona City Limits—announced our entrance into the college world. A sudden turn onto Huff Street took us slightly east past a small, calm lake with a walking path encircling it. College students walked, biked, and Rollerbladed all around the lake's trail. We had ignored the natural beauty as we drove farther from Anoka, but suddenly felt as if Winona was Minnesota's most picturesque city. We looked a block ahead on the right and Lonnie broke our sightseers' trance, "There it is!"

We were giddy with excitement and fear as we spotted the tall brick building that would be called home throughout our freshman year. Lonnie's nervous laughter was contagious, and all I could think about was the fact that I had been waiting for this moment all summer long. Lonnie pulled her car into a parking spot and we opened our doors simultaneously. We looked up at the tallest building in the city of Winona and smiled in awe. I had been assigned a second-floor room; poor Lonnie had to lug her stuff up to the sixth floor. Unpacking was definitely less convenient for Lonnie.

It would be days before we'd learn that the nickname of our new residence hall was "Virgin Towers" ... until spring, that is, when traditionally renamed "Thirteen Floors of Whores." I doubt if this information would have changed our overwhelming sense of pride as we carried our bags and baskets of belongings from the cars to our tiny dorm rooms.

We spent the next few hours unloading three cars stacked with stuff for two college girls. Tom and his girlfriend, Michelle, had volunteered to drive my black Ford Taurus, packed with clothes and Johnny Depp movie posters. My parents' car hauled my TV, VCR, and a menagerie of knickknacks and wall items for dorm room decorating. Within a few hours, everything was unpacked; my mauve bed sheets were accented by the black-and-white hand-knit cat blanket, which I placed across the foot of my bed. All of my fall clothes had been hung in my tiny closet. Here, I possessed about half the storage space that was in my bedroom at home.

"When it gets down in the single digits, I'll bring my winter jacket and sweaters from home," I said, ignoring my concern for the lack of winter storage.

My dad stood up from the bed, took a deep breath, and said, "Well, I suppose we'd better get going."

I didn't want them to go. The longest I had ever been away from them were those three nights during my seventh-grade hospital stay, and even then I had seen them daily.

My excitement from the day faded fast as I gave my father a hug, and then my mom. *I'm really not sure what I am going to do without them. We've had so much fun together, and they've helped me with everything.* I didn't want to leave my mom's embrace, but I was a college student now. I slowly released my arms from around her body ... she was clearly leaving this move up to me. Everyone said good-bye, and I closed the door behind them.

I limped to my bed, sat down, and looked at the empty space

across from me. My roommate would not arrive until after freshman orientation next week. Behind my closed door, I could hear girls' voices, along with their parents', coming and going through my hallway. Yet I had never felt so alone in my life. Like the cat pictured on my blanket, I curled up on my bed to rest. *A nap will help me keep the spasticity down. I have to meet some of these girls—I don't want my shaking to be the only thing they notice about me.*

No matter how hard I tried to fall asleep, it was not going to happen. I got up from the bed and took the elevator to the sixth floor to see how Lonnie was settling in.

The first week at Winona State was absolutely exhausting. The nights endlessly dragged on. I couldn't sleep due to the heat and a train that seemed to barrel through my room at least once an hour, its whistle screaming at me, "Wake up!" I hadn't experienced spasticity like that since my muscle transfer at age twelve. At least this time there was no pain. But without decent sleep at night, I wasn't able to walk at all during the day. I became dependent on my scooter.

At first, I felt really awkward using the scooter—thinking *everyone is looking at me.* Yet, after a couple of days, I grew to like my scooter and was really grateful for it.

Every day after our orientation class let out, Lonnie and I took a walk around Lake Winona. Lonnie either used Rollerblades or she walked, while I sat on my scooter in comfort. I joked with her, "My thumb gets so tired pushing this lever."

Over the next year, Lonnie and I walked around Lake Winona a couple times a week when the weather allowed. I made sure my scooter got plugged in nightly, so my batteries didn't die. We learned this the hard way in the spring. While Lonnie walked and I rode my scooter around the lake for the second day in a row, I realized I hadn't charged my battery. We were about three-quarters of the way around the lake when I noticed that my scooter was slowing down.

"Lonnie, the battery is almost dead. I don't know if I can make it back."

Lonnie assured me that it would make it. "Just keep pressing the lever until we get back to the dorm."

I held the lever in with my thumb, but my scooter slowed drastically, until it came to a complete stop.

"The battery's dead," I said turning my head toward Lonnie.

"Oh, God," Lonnie said, laughing. "I guess I'll have to push you."

Lonnie got behind my scooter and began pushing. After the three blocks back to Sheehan Hall, Lonnie wasn't laughing any longer. It took superhuman strength to push me up the incline to our dorm. As Lonnie pushed, I steered the scooter into the maintenance closet where I charged it every night. As soon as the scooter was plugged in, Lonnie plunged into one of the bright-orange cushioned chairs in the student lounge located on the first floor of the dorm, kitty-corner from my scooter's storage.

"That was a hard workout!" she giggled, and let out a big sigh of relief.

"I owe you. What if that would have happened while I was alone?" I was more grateful than Lonnie would know.

"Note to self, girl," she laughed again. "Charge it ... every night!" We laugh about this often—every time we reminisce about our college days.

I got into the groove of college life fairly fast. I made friends and enjoyed my classes, even the eight o'clocks. Since I was a morning person, I registered for 8:00 A.M. classes, Monday through Friday, and was typically done with my last class by noon every day. My roommate challenged this system since she was a night owl and slept late. That wouldn't have been a problem, except she snored like a bear in hibernation. Typically a nice person who would work around such things, this time I just couldn't adjust to her sleep habits. My mobility, as well as the use of my arms, was so impaired by my lack of sleep, something had to give.

I started to go to bed by 9:00 P.M. every night, so I could get in a good three hours of sleep before her snoring began. Every night, I would wake up to old-man snoring sounds coming from the other bed. At times, I turned to yell, "Stop snoring," but I knew it wouldn't do any good. She was hearing impaired and took out her hearing aids nightly. One time, I couldn't take it any longer. I threw a small pillow at her. She rolled over, and the snoring stopped long enough for me to attempt sleep again.

I complained to Lonnie about the excessive snoring. "I'm more and more exhausted! I'm starting to despise my roommate. She's crippling me—worse than I already am!"

Lonnie heard more than she probably wanted to know. "To make matters worse, she confides in me about things that I don't want to hear: warts, abortions, failing classes, and terrible boyfriends. I'm not sure how much more of this I can take."

"Why don't you say something? Speak up—let her know you want things to change," Lonnie advised me.

"It would all be bearable I suppose, if I wasn't so sleep-deprived," I admitted. "Luckily, she goes home every weekend, so I can get some survival sleep."

One Saturday evening, I was walking the block to the cafeteria when I was stopped by a classmate. "You're not using your scooter?" she inquired, as if something was wrong with me for walking.

I explained that since my roommate was gone for the weekend, I could get better sleep … "which helps my walking. I'm sure it doesn't make much sense, but this is how my life has always been. I get a good night's rest, and I get a good day of walking. If I don't get a full nine hours of sleep at night, my walking is limited. Then, I either have to take a nap, or give in to the scooter."

"Wow. You shouldn't have to put up with that," the girl replied before moving on.

Sunday always came too fast. I was back at it, sleeping with the chainsaw. *I'm not sure how much more my body can take.* I looked over at the person who is stealing my mobility little by little every night. In the shadows of our dark room, I saw round bumps that resembled her breasts. *That can't be so.* I squinted in the darkness to discover that indeed my roommate was spread eagle—her full frontal naked body on top of her twin bed. *Who does this? It can't be normal! Put some pajamas on, for Heaven's sake! I know this is college and everything, but can't she have a little modesty? How did I get stuck with her?*

She had told me that she didn't have many friends—now I knew why. *This has to end.* I complained to my friends about the boobs that I saw in the night. They, too, were shocked. It was at that moment that they all agreed, "You win. You have the worst roommate of us all. You need to do something."

Over Thanksgiving break, I had my neurology appointment with Dr. Anderson. As usual, he had me walk in the hall. He followed it up with a concerned look. He informed me that I was not walking as well as I used to.

"Are you getting rest at college?"

"No!" I announced. Then I explained that my roommate snored so loudly that "the only uninterrupted sleep I get is a three-hour stretch at the start of the night, if I beat her to bed." I followed with, "I try to take a nap every day, hoping to improve my walking for the afternoon. Sometimes this works."

"You need your own room." This time I was thankful for Dr. Anderson's blunt bedside manner.

I explained, "There are no more single rooms open in my residence hall."

"I'll take care of that." He explained that he would write a letter to the residence hall director as soon as I gave him the contact information.

"Get me that name and address. Things will change." He sounded so sure of this, I felt the stress from another sleepless night lifting. Just as he was leaving the exam room, he turned and said, "Now, get some sleep. You need sleep to survive. Everyone does."

Something was very different about this visit with Dr. Anderson. This was the first time I had felt he was on my side. Mom was right—she always said, "He is thinking of your best interests," even if I didn't notice it. *Thanks to him, I am going to get my own dorm room. I'm going to sleep! Normal sleep! Then, I'll be able to walk. Maybe I can use my scooter less ... maybe walk to my 8:00 A.M. classes.* I hadn't been able to do this in over a month. I was so excited when I left Dr. Anderson's that day!

I returned to school after the Thanksgiving break, and realized I was going to have to break the news to my roommate. I'd have to explain why I was getting my own room. The idea of having this conversation made me want to vomit. I didn't want to hurt her feelings. *Plus, I get the feeling she has low self-esteem—it makes this harder.* I bit the bullet and told her what Dr. Anderson had told me.

She felt bad that she had put this on me. I assured her, "It's okay—it's not your fault."

Two long weeks later, the hall director informed me that my new room was ready. "There wasn't a single dorm room available, so they turned the second floor study room into your dorm room."

It was the same size as my current dorm room. *Wow, it's twice the size of a single person dorm room.* As Lonnie helped me move all of my stuff down the hall, I was elated with the move. *I am going to get a good night's rest... on a weeknight!* Lonnie helped me move and set up, but at 8:55 P.M. she announced that she had to go.

"There's a new ER on tonight!"

I thanked her for her help, closed my single room door, and stared at the empty tan walls. I looked out my new window and silently thanked God for my great friend while noticing the view of the Sheehan Hall entrance. I spotted the cafeteria situated across the parking lot, and noticed some students on bikes and Rollerblades heading toward the lake trail. *I'm going to like it here. He pulled it off ... I can no longer say that Dr. Anderson hasn't helped me. This is a great room with a view.*

A Minor Major Change

I SURVIVED MY FRESHMAN YEAR, AND THEN MY FIRST SUM-
mer back home became an adventure I had not expected. By early
spring, I had sent out about a dozen cold contact letters to different
law firms in the Twin Cities, hoping to snag some paralegal experience for my resume before I went any further in my major. I got
one interview with a personal injury law firm and they hired me
as the summer gopher. I ran photocopies, fetched groceries (pop,
chocolate, and ibuprofen), and answered the phones while the receptionist went on break. The job paid well, but I was exhausted by
the end of every day. I was so fatigued from being on my feet for
most of my shift, I couldn't imagine doing this type of work for a
serious long-term career. The kicker was, each case that neared trial
date stirred up even more stress for the paralegals. As I observed
their work, I realized paralegal demands went far beyond my gopher
duties. I couldn't see any joy in a job that would ultimately prove too
demanding for me, physically and emotionally.

Thus, by midsummer, I not only hated my job, I felt the pressure
to rethink my entire college plan. I spent any free time searching for
a new major before I returned to Winona State University for my
second year of college.

*So, now what? I need a WSU course catalog. There has to be a major that
will lead to a job I can manage for more than one stressful summer.* The
public relations classes caught my attention and became my second
temporary major. The PR coursework seemed intriguing—maybe
even fun. *I've already registered for my fall classes so I can't change now.*

But they are general electives that will apply toward my undergrad require-ments. Looks like this will all work out!

The new major definitely started as the right fit for me. I received Bs or higher in the PR classes and enjoyed meeting some new students. Yet, fall of my junior year changed everything. I had to take Paul Lewiston's News Gathering class. I had a hard time watching him teach the course, let alone fulfill the assignments I often saw as ridiculous. He was the most arrogant person I had ever met.

Every day, just before he swaggered into class, we vented on how much we hated him, probably because we all feared he would fail us. The hardest part—he seemed to know this, and we were convinced that he enjoyed it.

I liked writing and did very well in my pre-req for News Gathering. However, we'd just gotten word that Professor Lewiston would be the only one teaching the course in the future. I had spent much of my time at WSU avoiding his classes, but there were no other options.

Throughout that next semester, I complained to my closest friends. "I have lost so much sleep over Lewiston's class, I am back to using my scooter morning, noon, and night." There was no physically good part to my day any longer, and I was definitely failing his class. I would never get a passing grade on a paper he assigned because, quite frankly, I refused to use the tactics he demanded for a story. In Lewiston's class each student was given a "beat." My beat was "professors," so although I could have been an incredible voice for issues like ADA, or other human interest topics, I was only allowed to write about WSU instructors. Lewiston wanted me to write "juicy" articles that would "raise eyebrows"—or at least his.

He wants me to wait outside a professor's home, in the bushes ... to watch and listen for good gossip? That's crazy. I wouldn't do that for two reasons: First, I felt it was morally wrong and, second, I physically couldn't accomplish this. My disability made this absurd, demeaning, and a deterrent to a passing grade. *I swear he smirks when he hands out each new assignment to me, knowing that it will lead to another failing grade.*

I literally began to feel sick every day as I gathered my things to go to his class. *It makes me ill that he enjoys seeing students sweat in his presence.* When my report card came in the mail with all Bs and one F, for News Gathering, I wasn't at all surprised, but I still fumed with tears in my eyes.

My parents had listened to me rant each week on the phone, and knew this class was making my life a living hell. Once the failure became reality, they agreed—I had to revisit the big questions again: *Do I transfer colleges? Or change my major?*

"I will never sit in one of his classes again," I made this clear to Mom and Dad. After lots of tears and discussions with my parents, I decided not to switch schools, but to consult the big book once again … and that search ironically landed me in my third and final undergraduate major: organizational communications.

My parents agreed with every point I made to defend wsu: "I really like Winona State. I have a lot of friends who are a great support system. I like the town and the other professors that have helped me out." There was no clear reason to transfer schools; I just had to avoid one arrogant instructor.

Nancy Dumke, the disability coordinator, was one of those helpful staff members who had supported me so much throughout my first two years at wsu. In fact, we had collaborated to work toward creating a more handicap-accessible campus. Opening the doors of campus buildings all on my own became our focus. When approaching each public building, ramps existed to accommodate scooters or wheelchairs. However, only a couple of the entrances had push-button door openers. For example, to get into the cafeteria, a building I frequented more than once a day, I had to scooter two blocks out of the way. First, the main doors did not have a curb-cut nearby, and secondly, the entrance lacked a push button for those times I arrived on my own.

I talked with Nancy about considering these accessibility changes, and she was thrilled to help me defend my suggestions when I made them to the school's administration. "This university will put money into accessibility needs as long as there's a current student telling them what is vital and essential for campus independence," Nancy shared.

The cold winters made me realize that I shouldn't have to go two blocks out of my way in below freezing temperatures to get into the cafeteria or the weight room. Nancy submitted my requests for push-button access for several of the buildings, but said that the board rejected my request for the buttons to be connected to levers that could be reached while still sitting on my scooter.

"What? I still have to get off my scooter to pull the doors open? What about future students who can't possibly leave their wheelchairs or their scooters without help? It seems a waste of time and money to do this halfway. It's like an accident waiting to happen," I explained my frustration with the decision.

"I agree. Let's make an appointment for you to talk directly to the man in charge of this. If you explain the design needed, I think he'll better understand your point of view. This will save the university time and money in the long run." Nancy encouraged me to pursue the best modification. She set up a time with the gentleman in charge, and I explained to him that my arms did not work like that of an able-bodied person.

"Unlike the other student currently at wsu who can't use her legs, but has normal use of her arms, I can't reach out and pull a door open. Plus, my scooter juts out a foot beyond my arm's reach, making it impossible to press a door button while sitting on the scooter. If I scoot up as closely as possible, the door will get stuck on the front of my scooter anyway. If I get off my scooter to walk over to a button placed flush on the side of the building, I am taking a chance of slipping on the ice in the winter." I did my best to show and tell him exactly why the buttons had to be placed away from the building.

Not long after our meeting, Nancy informed me that they would be placing the buttons on levers before the doors. We both felt victory, and Nancy said that this change would invite more students with physical disabilities to attend wsu.

Now that I knew I wanted to stay at wsu for the rest of my college education, I was ready to tackle my new major.

My very first Intro to Speech class graded students on two exams and four speeches. The thought of speaking in front of twenty of my college peers took me back to the agoraphobia episode of eleventh grade. This time, however, I was on my own to pick my topic, gather information, and prepare to face the room full of listeners. There was no turning back with communications as my major. My first speech had to be planned, practiced, and executed within two weeks. Professor Linton had students sign up for a time slot for each speech, so I placed my name at the top of this list for speech number one. *I want to go first, so I can get it over with and not compare myself to others that go before me.*

For the next two weeks, I researched my topic: adaptations for disabilities. The night before my big speech, I felt like I might vomit. *Why am I having so much trouble remembering my speech? I can't hold note cards in these shaky hands.* I could feel my nerves getting the best of me. *Maybe I should call the professor and tell him I'm sick, which would not be a lie.* At the same time, I knew that eventually I had to give this speech, and more importantly, I had to conquer this performance anxiety. I remembered the trick my instructor shared that had worked for him for years. I walked to the mirror that hung in my small dorm closet.

I faced the frightened girl staring back at me and began my speech.

"Imagine an entire generation of polio victims who didn't attend college because they simply couldn't get up the stairs to the university's library ... or, a girl with MS who loved movies, but quit going because her local theater, with concrete steps and narrow walkways, was impossible to navigate from a wheelchair ... or a man who re-trained himself to work after an accident, but lost his job anyway when the employer decided the work station required too many modifications ... these are the stories that helped write the ADA legislation ... these are the reasons to fight for the adaptations and modifications needed for individuals with disabilities—yes, even on this very campus. Sure, the Americans with Disabilities Act of 1990 quote 'prohibits discrimination and ensures equal opportunity for persons with disabilities in employment, state and local government services, public accommodations, commercial facilities, and transportation' unquote. Yet, how can this law ensure the rights of disabled Americans if access to public buildings remains the number one obstacle for citizens with debilitating conditions?"

My confidence grew as I slowly spoke, enunciating every single word in front of that mirror. I could feel it … these words were important. I honestly wanted to share them with others—make people listen to something I felt passionate about. After delivering my speech two more times to the young woman in the mirror, I brushed my teeth and crawled into bed to await the clock's read-out of 7:00 A.M.

The next morning, I arrived to speech class thirty minutes early, hoping that this would tame my nerves. When I walked in, I was surprised to find another student sitting all alone at a desk. He was my age and had thick auburn hair.

"Hey," he said with a forced smile.

"Hi," I replied back, trying not to sound too astonished that someone had beaten me into the room.

Clearly, I had met a student with a worse case of stage fright than mine.

"I'm Trevor," I recall his deep voice, but immediately forgot his name as my own nerves kicked in again. We chatted about wanting to get the first speech over … 8:00 A.M. couldn't come soon enough. Then other students began trickling in.

"Good luck—you'll do great." This was my cue to focus on the long walk up to the front of this rather standard classroom … any room seemed large and intimidating when a speech grade was on the line.

"Thanks," I said, grateful for the encouraging words. "Good luck to you too."

"Jean Sharon." I think I jumped off my seat when I heard my name called. *That's me! Oh, yeah, I signed up to go first!* I was thankful that the podium had not been banned this time, and grateful for some attentive-looking listeners. I left that class with a gratified feeling that more speeches could be conquered—as long as Paul Lewiston didn't teach the class.

Steve One and Steve Two

EMMA AND I LOUNGED IN HER DORM ROOM NOT LONG AFTER I had survived that first speech. Suddenly, Samantha barged into the room—her face red with embarrassment. She had just let herself into one of the guy's dorm rooms to measure the space for carpeting. Her friend Troy, who was entering Winona State as a freshman, and would arrive in a few days, had asked Samantha to get precise numbers for him.

"I can't believe I went there to measure for carpet in a room that already had it! I can only imagine what his roommate thinks."

"There was a guy in there? What did he look like?" I asked, leaning forward and smiling with interest.

"Oh, you would really like him," she smiled, while wiping the sweat from her forehead.

The September heat in Sheehan Hall is torture without the coolness of an air conditioner. Samantha sat down on the worn gray love seat, hugging her water bottle.

"He wasn't wearing a shirt," Samantha seemed mortified, which made Emma laugh. "You would like his chest," Samantha directed this comment to me. "It's really muscular and there isn't any hair on it."

By this point in our college lives, Samantha and Emma knew me well. They understood everything about me … my physical limitations, my desire to do well in my new major, *and* my interest in shirtless guys.

Both girls encouraged my habit of flirting, I think because deep down they knew I could never take it further. Flirting at school was rather easy for me, likely because there was no expectation for things to go beyond the superficial small talk. Ironically, when I did have a true interest in someone, I clammed up and hardly said a word, which wasn't very often. I believed that no one from college could reciprocate my genuine interest. Let's just say I picked up on a pattern. If a guy's first impression of me was standing or walking, he never saw me as dating material. On the other hand, if his first glimpse of me was at a table in the cafeteria or library, that same guy might actually strike up a conversation—and sometimes a flirtatious one at that. Unfortunately, when he realized that I could barely walk, his interest faded to a "nice meeting you" or a "see ya around" departure.

I understood this: *It is going to take a really special man to want to date a girl with life-altering physical limitations. The guy I end up dating won't be able to go running, walking, or swimming or play sports with me.* Mom always said this is precisely why I would end up with "the nicest one of all." At the start of my junior year, the activities that most couples hoped to do made up a rather short list when I was involved.

I could sense that Samantha was flustered about the new guy. "He must be really cute," I said. "Tell me what he said when you walked in on him … "

I soon met Steve—the new guy with the already-carpeted dorm room. Samantha had every right to be embarrassed and flustered when she saw him. He had everything that I am physically attracted to in a guy: broad shoulders, a beefed-up chest, dark brown hair, and big brown eyes that looked right at you when you spoke. The best part—he was six feet seven, standing a whole foot taller than me. Even his voice was sexy. He didn't say a lot, but when he did, I listened intently. I usually gave guys a lot of attention by looking their way or giving them a big smile, but for some reason, when Steve looked me in the eye, I couldn't look back.

Steve is out of my league and no matter how attractive I find him, I know it's not possible for him to feel the same way about me. Scholarship basket-

ball players are not interested in girls who use a scooter to get to class. It's too bad, because he is really good-looking.

Steve spent plenty of time with our group. Emma, Samantha, Troy, Steve, and I ate dinner together in the cafeteria almost every night. *I think Troy likes Emma. He has this intense look when she speaks— like he wants to hear every word she says. I'm sure that it's just a matter of time before they start dating.* Emma was one of those girls that guys really liked. Her beautiful blonde hair and big blue eyes lit up when she smiled. She was a fun, spirited girl who talked and laughed as much as I did.

As I predicted, Troy and Emma started dating. I was happy for her, except I really wanted something like that as well. No one had ever shown any interest in me, besides friendship. *I'm not really sure what that would be like. But I'd like to find out someday. It would be wonderful to watch television with a guy and have him put his arm around me . . . and put his hand on my hand . . . and run his thumb on the back of my hand.* Obviously, I had plenty of time to watch other couples.

I told my mom that I really thought I'd be alone forever: "It's not possible for a guy to want to be with me."

She assured me again, "You will end up with the nicest one of all."

It would be false to say that no one was ever interested in me. During my freshman year, a boy named Amir bugged me for months to go out with him. I just wasn't attracted to him. He was shorter than me, for one thing, and I had some trouble understanding his Middle Eastern dialect. I did finally go out with him, after many invitations. But I could tell it wasn't going to work.

I agreed to go to dinner off-campus one night. When we got to the restaurant, many of the older patrons stared at us, or should I say, me. Their eyes followed my limp from the hostess podium all the way to our booth. I'm used to this, but Amir was not.

"This is really rude—why would people just stare at you because of your walk?"

I laughed and said, "They're just staring because we're so good-looking." Nothing. Amir had the same irritated expression, and I think the whole thing bothered him the rest of the evening.

Needless to say, Amir and I didn't go out on a date ever again. However, we still got together occasionally when our old college group reunited. He would look at me and tell me I was still so pretty. I would wait for the line I heard over and over from him, back in the dorm, with that unique Middle Eastern dialect: "I really want to kiss your lips."

The first time I heard this, a million thoughts raced through my head: *I'm nineteen years old and I've never experienced a kiss. I'm not sure that I ever will have a first kiss, or make love with someone who really loves me for me. I don't believe that I will ever know what it's like to have someone show real feelings for me.*

This was a lot to process while Amir waited for permission to kiss me. I wanted so badly for someone to love the person I was on the inside, as well as my clumsy legs, and my helpless hands. At that moment, I was positive that I would die without experiencing any kind of love from a man.

"Thanks. But, I'm not kissing you," I said in my blunt yet playful way—false hope for Amir to try again … and again.

* * *

As was true for most campus students, the dorm bed often became the sofa for social visits and TV watching. So, a few days later, Amir and I plopped down on my bed for some mindless TV and small talk. Out of nowhere, Amir stopped talking and began to gawk at me.

"What?" I stated, sensing his silent stare.

"I really want to kiss you," he informed me while dragging both of his hands through his black curly hair. *Hmm … I've heard this line before.*

The fact that I had turned this offer down on a previous night did not make this an easy decision. All the same thoughts came rushing back: *I've never been kissed. No one has ever thought about kissing me. This may be my only chance to be kissed. I'm not excited to kiss him, but then again, this may be my only shot before I die … and I plan to live a long life. I just don't foresee anyone else ever showing any interest in kissing me in my future. Okay. There has to be a way that I can let him kiss me without him thinking that I want to kiss him.*

115

"I'll let you kiss me if you can tell me my birthday," I stated with a smirk.

He grinned at me, then gently pushed me back and straddled my hips. He clearly knew he had a chance, but I also saw the calendar clicking away in his mind.

He doesn't remember my birthday!

I saw in his eyes that he really wanted to kiss me, but the stress of remembering my birthday was getting to him.

"Okay. It's June 20."

"Nope," I gloated, but felt a little disappointment at the same time.

"July 10?"

"Well, at least you have the right month," I hinted.

"Aha! It's July 20, isn't it?!" He took such pride in his guess.

"Wow. Only three tries," I said sarcastically.

Amir leaned down to kiss me, and I have to say, it was everything a kiss should *not* be! His tongue rammed down my throat. It felt like I was tolerating a medical procedure with a foreign instrument searching for a problem in my throat—trying to pinpoint something that wasn't even there. When he finally leaned back and took his hips off of mine, I felt compelled to wipe the saliva from my mouth.

He said good-bye and left. I don't even recall if he appeared satisfied, or disappointed. All I remember was that I had hoped for a first kiss better than this. *Maybe I was pushing it ... I might have been better off dying without that.*

That year, Valentine's Day at Winona State fell on a Friday. Kim and I sat in the commons area of Sheehan Hall selling roses to benefit the Inter Residence Hall Council. There wasn't much going on and we hadn't sold very many flowers. I saw Steve walk in using crutches, so I waved him over.

"What are you doing here?" I said, smiling. I knew he had scheduled some kind of procedure ... something to do with part of a quad muscle that had calcified and had to be removed.

"Oh," he sighed. "My truck was towed while I had my surgery."

"What? That stinks. Do you need some help getting it back? I can take you to pick it up," I offered.

"That would be great … can you take me tomorrow morning?"

"No problem," I assured him.

We made small talk about the flowers and I introduced Kim to Steve. Kim and her smile sat alongside me, illuminating the lobby. It was clear that she thought Steve was an attractive guy.

"What are your plans for dinner tonight?" Steve asked me. Our group typically ate together in the campus cafeteria, but given it was Valentine's Day, Emma and Troy planned to go out, and Samantha had different plans with other friends as well.

"Uh, I don't know. Do you want to meet in the cafeteria?" I asked, uncertain of what his thoughts were. *Why does Valentine's Day have to complicate things? We're just two friends who happen to be the opposite sex, and eat dinner together almost every night.*

"No. Would you want to come to my place? We could order a pizza tonight?" he asked me.

"Okay," I answered, with a little surprise in my voice.

Steve said to come at six—he'd order the pizza then. He turned and walked out of the dorm lobby. Kim and I watched as the tall glass door swung shut behind him.

"You've got a date!" Kim squealed as she turned more in my direction.

"No, I don't," I stated, then straightened the red roses in the vase in front of me. "Steve and I are just friends."

"I don't care what you say," Kim insisted. "You're going over there for pizza on a Friday night and it's Valentine's Day. That's a date."

There was nothing I could say to make it clear this was not a date. "Steve and I are just friends who happen to eat dinner together. The only difference tonight is, none of our other friends can join us." Although I don't think Kim was convinced that this was a non-date pizza event, I never gave it another thought.

Not exactly an exotic culinary choice, but pizza in Steve's room represented a change in our dining experience. For three straight years, I predictably consumed almost all of my nutrition from wsu's campus dining hall. Every morning, I carried my breakfast tray to my table. By lunch, searching out the same table, I carried my tray about half the time. By evening dinner, however, I needed help, which generally came from a work-study student carrying my tray to that same rear table. The day's demands gradually sucked the strength right out of my limbs. Although eating off-campus sometimes sounded fun, the dining hall was an apt and reliable setting for me.

Always cognizant of the need to pace myself, I parked my scooter by the nearest cafeteria door. Efficiency became intuitive. Without much thought, I seemed to always find the shortest route from point A to point B. *So what if this put me at the cafeteria table closest to the waste conveyor belt ... and the garbage cans?* My scooter was parked directly outside this waste-area exit. Throughout my freshman year, I could count on Angie and Lonnie, and perhaps their roommates, to join me at my table in the back.

"Why do you think they always put us by the garbage?" Lonnie finally asked one day. I laughed so hard, and then explained to her that I had *chosen* this table. "No one stuck me here." Lonnie, Angie, and I laughed and reminisced so much at that table.

It goes without saying that I would not be the person I am today without Angie and Lonnie. Our friendships continued long after I moved from their neighborhood at three years old. We played a lot as kids, reunited when Winona emerged as our mutual yet unplanned college choice, then later in our adult lives we started up again with playdates for our own children. I have always been able to be myself around them and their families. When I think of my friendships with these two women, I feel so thankful that they never gave in to the pressure of treating me differently during those early years—especially in junior high. When so many kids either ignored me or teased me, they never stopped being my friend. It's possible that they experienced an internal dilemma over their friendship with me. I don't know, and I wouldn't have blamed them if they debated this. It would have been difficult to befriend someone who is so different from everyone else. I'm not going to dwell on this because they never showed any concern for it in front of me, which means the world to me. Their unconditional friendships remain such an important part of my life.

Although most of our childhood adventures replayed at some

point during those campus meals our freshman year, one favorite recurring story became our favorite to share. It happened when Angie and I were about seven ... when she had come with my family to a campground that had horse trails.

The last thing I wanted to do on a camping trip was horseback ride. Everyone has one bad experience on a horse, and mine occurred while riding with my brothers the previous summer. I had ended up on the underside of an animal intent upon passing my brothers' horses. I repeated to Angie, "I can't ride a horse ... I'm gonna fall off like last year."

Angie became very encouraging, "You won't fall off, Jean. You can do it." Angie wanted to go horseback riding more than anything else on this camping trip. I did not want to let her down, so I gave in ... "Okay, we can go."

Angie and I each got our own adult horse. My brothers led the pack, while Angie followed behind me. Everything started out fine. My horse walked slowly while I held onto the knob of the saddle. Then, an instant replay of last summer's event kicked in ... Mike's horse began to run and Tom's followed suit. My horse took the hint and ran after them. I had no control or power to stop, and as I bounced up and down on my horse, my saddle began slowly sliding to the right. In no time, the saddle had moved to the belly side of the horse and I held onto it with all my strength. I could hear Angie screaming, "Hang on, Jean! Don't let go of the horse!" At the same moment, a strange man on a horse came running next to me.

"Let go!" he yelled at me.

I continued to hold on for dear life. *If he thinks I'm going to let go and risk being trampled, he's crazy.*

"Let go!" he yelled again. "You have to let go. The horse won't step on you."

At that moment, I knew I had to trust this man. I couldn't ride into the night like this. I let go. As I hit the dirt-covered ground, the horse kept running after my brothers, and Angie's horse followed. I stood up, brushed the dirt off the knees of my jeans, and trudged back to the starting point. When Angie reappeared, I could see so much concern in her big blue eyes.

"Are you okay, Jean?" she asked, getting off of her horse.

"Yeah, but I'm never doing that again," I answered with authority.

It's been over twenty-five years since that happened and Angie and I can talk about it as though it happened yesterday. We usually laugh so hard when we share the details of this, I don't know how anyone listening can hear a word we're saying ... yet Lonnie seems able to narrate it now.

Mealtime continued to be a highlight of my days at Winona State. But, by year two, Lonnie had transferred to St. Cloud State and Angie had moved off campus. Starting my sophomore year, I ate most of my meals with Emma, Samantha, and Troy, and by the month of February, with Steve. I will be forever grateful for the friendships and memories created by those mealtime gatherings in our college dining hall.

At 6:00 P.M. that Valentine's Day, I put on my black winter coat and gloves, locked my dorm room door, and slowly dragged my left leg down the flight of stairs to my scooter, parked in storage. I smiled at the two security guards at the main entrance as I pushed the handicap button that opened the door to the world outside of Sheehan Hall.

All alone, I could turn the accelerator dial to the picture of the rabbit on my scooter to speed along a little faster than usual. I coasted down the ramp, then drove across the parking lot, grateful to whiz by the cafeteria for something different that night. Steve's dorm didn't have an accessible door, so I parked my scooter just outside his old brick building. I pulled the key from the scooter and placed it in my coat pocket, knowing someone may try to prank me by moving it ... it had happened before. I slowly opened the door and felt the welcome warmth of Steve's dorm lobby on my face and hands. I took a few steps down the hall to the third door on the left, and knocked.

Steve opened the door, all smiles. My eyes went directly to his face, but lowered slowly down all six and a half feet of this lean athlete, until the brown carpet on the floor caught my eye. I laughed on the inside, thinking of Samantha just a few months prior to this night. *Yes, there's carpet in this room.* I took a seat on the couch that nestled under the lofted bunk. We made small talk for a while. Then Steve called to order a large pizza with everything on it.

I was able to eat my pizza at ease, since the nap I took that afternoon recharged my body. My arms, hands, and fingers cooperated, unlike most Friday nights when I was wiped from a long week.

When dinner was over, Steve and I decided to watch a movie ... an 80s favorite for both of us—*Hoosiers.*

Steve started the movie and turned off the lights, leaving just the slight glow from the television and his white holiday lights left up after Christmas. I eased down to the floor to let my back rest on the base of the couch.

"You can sit on the couch if you want," Steve stated, looking down on the floor.

"Oh, no, thanks. I like stretching out on the floor," I replied, straightening my legs on the carpet.

Steve nodded his head, and moved to sit on the floor next to me, leaving a foot of flooring between us.

Halfway into the movie, the Christmas lights went out. The room became dark with the exception of the streetlights shining in through the window. Just as fast as they went out, they flickered back on. I turned to face Steve. *Was I the only one to notice this?* We smiled at one another and turned our attention back to Gene Hackman coaching the basketball team to victory.

As the film credits rolled up the television screen, I climbed to my feet and put on my jacket. *It's time for me to go. Troy will bring Emma back here at any time and I really don't want to deal with them.* I knew that this evening was not a date, but I could predict Emma's silly inquiries if she and Troy thought we made out all night.

"So, how was the movie?" she would ask. "Or maybe you didn't get to it. That's okay. It is Valentine's Day after all." They would laugh, Steve and I would look awkwardly at each other ... it just wasn't worth lingering in his room any longer.

* * *

The following Friday, with my bridesmaid's dress in hand, I left for Rochester to attend my brother Tom's wedding. After dating Michelle for four years, Tom decided to tie the knot. *I have been looking forward to this weekend for months! I can see a lot of family—and Steve.* I really enjoyed being in the company of Tom's best friend, Steve. Yes, another Steve!

Tom and Steve had been tolerating my pleas to join their fun since junior high. In high school—they were college boys by then—I often tagged along to weekend movies. Sometime during my freshman year, things seemed to have changed between Steve and me. We started teasing and flirting every time we got together. I'm not really sure how or why things changed. All I know is that I had a lot of fun when I was with him, and eventually thought of him as more than my brother's best friend. I knew I had feelings for him, and I sensed that this was mutual. In fact, the last time we were alone, we made a pact that if neither one of us was married by the year 2000,

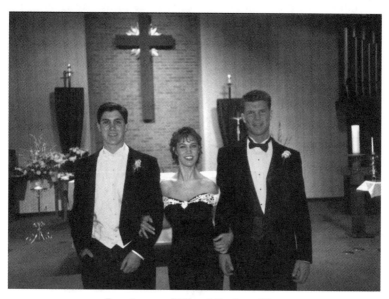

Tom, Jean, and Mike at Tom's wedding

we would marry each other. There was only one problem: *This* Steve had a girlfriend.

I predicted a breakup, which gave me hope that Steve would be available soon. Whenever Tom, Steve, and I hung out together, Steve spent most of the time complaining about her.

"Dump her," Tom would advise. But I was convinced that Steve lacked the confidence to do something so drastic.

The morning of Tom's wedding, Mom and I got our hair done. The stylist curled all of my hair and put it up, then left my bangs to fall softly across my forehead. *I love it!* Afterward, we headed back to the hotel and I put on the sexy navy strapless dress that Michelle had picked out for her bridesmaids. I looked in the mirror and was honestly stunned at all of my curves—they were showing in just the right places. This was *not* my normal attire, and I wondered how my family would react to my appearance. Most had never seen me in a dress before.

"Jean, it's time to go," I heard my dad call from the other side of the bathroom door. I grabbed my jacket, but in the hotel corridor, I was greeted by my other brother's girlfriend, Janel.

"Let me do your makeup, Jean," Janel smiled, pulling me into her hotel room.

"Dad says we have to go," I resisted her.

"I can do it really fast!" Janel stated.

Suddenly, I was pinned up against the wall of Janel's room while she applied foundation to my face. I had never worn makeup in my life, so I really didn't know if I welcomed this opportunity so late in the morning of my brother's wedding day. *What if I don't like this? What if I look horrible? Like a clown?* She took a couple more items out of her bag of tricks, and in a matter of two minutes, she urged me to turn and face the mirror.

My mouth fell open, and for the first time, I was speechless. *I'm not sure who this girl is looking back at me. She's beautiful.* I had never looked like this in my life!

Excited to be a part of the wedding, I arrived at the church for pictures. My nerves sent a strong message: *Take the stairs to the sanc-*

tuary slowly … especially with these dress shoes on. At school, I lived in sneakers. It's common to have gowns altered, but I also had my shoes changed by adding a strap to secure my heels. Even with this added support, I took careful steps to find the wedding party.

I spied Tom near the sanctuary, standing with his three friends, Kip, Blake … and Steve. I felt a little uneasy approaching them, ready for the teasing to begin since I was all "dolled up," as the men in my family often called it. I took a deep breath and made my clumsy advance up the aisle, although I moved as gracefully as possible. I'm convinced that they heard my staggered, heavy steps because all three men turned their heads to look in my direction simultaneously. The looks on their faces resembled that of my own just an hour before, as I spotted myself in the hotel mirror. I sensed that all three shared the same thought—that I was no longer Tom's little sister.

A couple hours later, Steve and I were standing next to one another, waiting to walk down the aisle together. Logically, I was matched up with Steve because I was the tallest bridesmaid, and he was the tallest groomsman at six feet four. I linked my shaking arm in his, as Steve assured me that I had nothing to be nervous about.

"We'll get you down the aisle safely." I was so grateful that my groomsman had known me for most of my life. I trusted Steve with every fiber of my being.

The director gestured us to start our walk down the aisle. Steve turned to me and whispered, "This is our dry run for the year 2000."

With his words swimming in my head, I followed his lead down the aisle, my smile beaming the entire way. *Maybe it is possible that there is someone out there who can love me completely. Is it possible that he's beside me right now?*

I had a difficult time staying focused on the wedding. All I thought about was Steve, and every time I looked over at him, our eyes met. *I don't think he's paying much attention to the ceremony either. I'm not sure, but I think my life has changed today.*

At the reception, I couldn't stop thinking about Steve. *I need to tell him how I really feel. I'll be taking a huge risk, but I fear that he's too shy to ever tell me how he feels.* I couldn't let this thought go, especially after his comment.

Suddenly, the DJ announced that the bridal party should take the floor for a slow dance. *Are you kidding me? I can hardly stand on my own two feet, much less move with someone else leading.*

Greeted by Steve, I reluctantly walked onto the dance floor. My shaking launched me back to reality, yet Steve assured me with quiet words that we'd be okay. "One slow dance—you'll be fine." We talked about the day's events, but all I thought about was how I truly wanted to be his girlfriend, despite the fact that Steve's actual girl-friend stood a few feet away as she observed our entire dance.

While Tom and my new sister-in-law slowly danced by us, I picked up on Michelle's sneaky cues. Her commands to declare my feelings to Steve came camouflaged in less-than-subtle body language.

Now! Michelle's eyes ordered. *He has you around the waist . . . he's leaning down to hear your every word . . . tell him now!*

My heart raced and my palms sweated, like a movie cliché played out on the bridesmaid's dance floor. I looked up at Steve.

"I need to tell you something, but I'm really nervous."

"What?" he said with the first serious face I had seen all evening. "You can tell me anything."

Wow—that makes me feel safe . . . he must feel the same way.

"I have feelings for you," I whispered, praying that he heard me because I didn't know if my mouth could ever form those words again.

"I feel the same way," he whispered back.

I could feel that he had tightened his grip on me ever so slightly. *I shared my deepest thought with him and I didn't get shot down.* Thoughts of never having a relationship—of never having a man look at me in a desirable way—came racing back to me. *This is amazing.* I relished the moment . . . then . . .

"But, I have a girlfriend," he said with sad eyes. He informed me that he hadn't broken up with her yet, and he wasn't going to cheat on someone. Steve assured me that he intended to end the relationship soon, ". . . and then we can be together." As if on cue, the song ended.

I spent the rest of the night mingling with all of the guests, but my mind was on Steve. Then, Steve's girlfriend approached me.

"I'd like to talk to you as soon as you get a chance."

Oh, dear Lord, what does she know? An hour later she sat down beside me.

"I can see why Steve likes you," she lowered her head. "You're beautiful." She talked to me for a few minutes, but I couldn't concentrate on anything she said. "I see how he looks at you." Clearly she saw the attraction, but she didn't seem to know what I told Steve. I felt like a horrible person. *They are going to break up soon and it's all my fault.* She told me goodbye, got up, and moved away from the table.

The reception had come to an end and I took a seat at a table in the back of the hall. Steve approached me to tell me that he and Lilly were leaving.

"I can't break up with her tonight." This matter-of-fact comment should be my final let-down for the evening.

But then he placed his hand on mine. "We will end up together. Maybe not right away, but it will work out in the end," he squeezed my hand, turned, and walked out the door, leaving me all by myself.

I know that Steve likes me, but he doesn't have enough of a backbone to break up with his girlfriend. Since the wedding, we began e-mailing one another, which was a lot of fun. It gave me something to look forward to at the end of the day. We didn't talk about much other than school, and I hadn't brought up my feelings to him again. Yet, when I received a photo from my mom of Steve and me standing together at the wedding, I thought we looked really cute together. *I still can't believe that I looked that good!* I decided to mail the photo to Steve with a letter. I didn't say anything about dating, but kept it at, "We look good together."

As I watched TV alone in my tiny dorm room on a Saturday evening, I thought how I would love it if Steve would call me. Around 9:00 P.M., my phone rang. I silently prayed, "Please, be Steve."

"Hello," I said into my standard, white dorm phone.

"Hello, Miss Jean," I listened to the voice I so desperately wanted to hear.

We made small talk for a while, and then he mentioned my letter and the photo that I had sent.

"My friends saw our picture and couldn't believe how beautiful 'Taurus Woman' was."

He knew he had to clarify this. "'Taurus Woman'—that's you. You drive a Ford Taurus, right? My friends can't believe that you like me, and they think I should dump Lilly."

I politely told him that he had smart friends. Then, I asked if he had any intention of breaking up with her in the near future.

"I did break up with her." My heart jumped with excitement. "But, she begged me to take her back … so I did."

I didn't even know how to respond to this. My spirit was deflated just as fast as it was filled with hope. *I really like this guy, but he must not feel as strongly as I do. If he can't even break up with a girl he does nothing but complain about, we don't have a chance.*

We made small talk for a little while longer as he assured me this would "all work out in the end." *I don't know how he can say this. Steve, you might very well be the only person who thinks we have a chance of being together someday. Because right now, I have my doubts …*

More than Meals with Steve

I spent a wonderful spring break in Fort Lauderdale, Florida, with Mom and Dad. Nearly all of my time was spent soaking up the sun in my hot-pink Speedo bikini. My olive skin was five shades darker than the Minnesota pasty white I left behind at the Minneapolis airport just one week earlier.

As we flew home on Delta, my parents and I were seated in the exit row, which Dad liked since it provided some extra legroom. But as we were taxiing on the runway before takeoff, the flight attendant approached me.

"You seemed to have some difficulty walking onto the plane. Is everything okay?"

I told her that I was fine and that it was just a muscle disorder.

"I'm going to have to ask you to sit in a different row during takeoff and landing due to the safety and security of the other passengers." She went on to explain that I would not be able to do the necessary actions if, Heaven forbid, we experienced a crash.

I understood. A few extra responsibilities, however hypothetical, accompanied the extra legroom for these seats. I waved goodbye to my folks, and followed the aircrew worker to a different row.

"If the plane crashes, I don't think it will really matter who's sitting there," I said as I glanced back to my abandoned seat. "We'll all be dead." I laughed at my candid remark, and the flight attendant flashed a brief smile. I think she had heard that one before.

Shortly after the plane landed, my dad received a call on his cell phone. He turned to me and stated, "Tom and Michelle want to know if you can come to dinner tonight."

I knew what this was. *Dinner, sure ... plus an invitation for Steve to join us.* I was actually excited about the setup. "Yes! Tell them I can come ... let's find our luggage and get going!"

An hour later, I was knocking on Tom's door. Three of us prepared to sit down to dinner at a table that was clearly set for four.

"Steve's on his way," Michelle smiled at me.

I felt the anticipation of something special, but then again, feared this was going to be the same event I had been living over and over since Tom and Michelle's wedding. *He'll tell me how much he likes me ... but he's still got a girlfriend ... and he's not a cheater.*

I recalled the letter I sent him just a couple weeks before our spring break trip. I told him, "I'm not going to wait around forever." *If he wants to date me great, but I will not be led on, then have to wait for him.* Suddenly, my bold words in the letter gave me a wave of fear that I had been too forward.

When Steve arrived, we ate spaghetti and garlic bread, and our meal was filled with great conversation and lots of laughs. Tom and Michelle, a very happy couple, made me feel welcome—like I was a friend, not just a little sister.

After dinner, we visited over our dessert. Then Steve noticed it was dark outside. He looked at his watch and said, "I'd better get going." He turned to me and asked, "Do you need a ride?"

"Sure." I told him that Tom could give me a ride, but this would save him the trip.

Sounding cold, he replied, "It's not a big deal. Your parents' house is close to mine." Like I needed this information ...

I could tell he was different. *He's not being warm and inviting. I've never seen this side of him before.* I crawled into his gray Chevy pickup, very similar to Tall Steve's truck, from college.

I noticed that in my mind I had been referring to each of the Steves as "Tall Steve" or "Short Steve." I laughed to myself since they both were very tall, each standing about six and a half feet. For some reason, I no longer wanted to talk to Short Steve, so I stared out the passenger window as we pulled away from my brother's place.

"Well, Miss Jean, I got your letter."

Here it comes. I don't even want to have this discussion. He's been aloof and uninvolved for most of the evening.

"I told you that I'm not going to cheat on Lilly," he said, looking directly at me. Light radiated from the street lamp as he pulled up to a stop sign.

"I never asked you to cheat on her," I shot back, with irritation on my face and coldness in my voice. "I don't want to date you if you're seeing someone else." With that, I turned away and looked out the passenger side window. We were nearing my neighborhood. *Soon this conversation will be over—and so will my chance of ever dating Steve.* Anger and sadness prompted my next words.

"Steve, you are not the only guy. I will not sit at home and wait around for you." We were in my driveway. I felt for the door handle.

"You're dating?" his blue eyes widened with surprise.

"Yes," I looked back intently at him. "In fact, his name is Steve. I have to call one of you Tall Steve and the other Short Steve to keep the two of you straight."

With a smug grin on his face, he replied, "So, I'm Tall Steve to you?"

"No!" I stated, smugly. "You're Short Steve. The other Steve is six seven."

At this point, my body is beginning to boil, although I try not to shake. *He is so full of himself. I really think he believes that I will be here forever.* Then, sadly, I wonder if it is because he thinks no one else could find me attractive? I had spoken to God about this several times in the past and had accepted that I was destined to be alone forever. Sure, I wanted a husband and children, but if I wasn't able to find a caring person who could endure a life of challenges, that would have to be okay. I could still live a happy life. A life that God had mapped out for me.

"Have you been kissing any of these guys?" For the first time, I detected a little jealousy on his face and in his voice. Yet, this was a concerned look. His eyes had lost the fight in them.

Calmly, I responded, "I'd say they are more like kissing friends." I can't believe that I said this! I've never even come close to kissing Tall Steve. On the other hand, Short Steve needs to understand that I won't be here waiting forever. I may never officially *date* again, but that doesn't mean that I have to be treated like some desperate woman—although, that's exactly how all of this made me feel.

"I hope you're not sleeping with these guys," he said, looking me straight in the eye.

I might be able to lie about kissing a guy, but I could never have said I was sleeping with someone when I wasn't. My values and morals were in conflict with that on so many levels. I had always said that I would wait until marriage for that kind of relationship, and I didn't plan on changing that part of my life just out of anger.

"Of course not," I said to him.

"Jean, I know that you're not going to wait around for me and I fear that one day I'll come for you and you'll be with someone else. Then I'll have to fight to get you back." His anger had melted. He said this in a calm, almost sad way.

I remained silent to that and began opening my door.

"Do you need me to walk you to the door?"

"No, I can manage just fine," I said as the anger turned to hurt.

"I didn't mean it like that."

"I know. Can I give you a hug goodbye?" I asked, knowing that this was my last time with him.

"I'm not going to kiss you."

"I know," I said with much irritation in my voice. *How can he be that arrogant? This is not the guy I knew before. I've lost my friend Steve forever.*

I leaned over and lightly gave him a hug. I exited the truck, then stopped before shutting the door to whisper "goodbye," knowing that no matter what this was between Steve and me, the fun—the suspense of what it might have been, is over. And the friendship that had developed over years of being the tagalong sister will never be the same.

I walked to the front door of the house as quickly as I could; the cold hit my face with each struggling step. I wasn't sure what saddened me more—knowing that I would never date Steve or believing that he was my only shot at love, marriage, and kids.

* * *

Two years of breaking bread with the best group of friends I could ever ask for made me grateful for my life at Winona State. I am not overstating how important mealtime was—the highlight of my day. Where would I have been without Emma, Troy, Samantha, and Steve? Not one of them was bothered by my difficulty with walking, or my use of the scooter to get around campus. Even Friday night barhopping, once I turned twenty-one, was an inclusive event. These friends would not leave me home alone. At times, Emma heard me vent my spastic diplegia frustrations, but honestly, life just moved forward, so there wasn't much talk about it. My friends seemed to understand my different way of doing things, and accepted me for who I was. That's why, when disagreements arose between some of my inner group, I felt little control over the inevitable—things were about to change. Essentially, our pack was fated to split up.

Emma spent all of her time with Troy. Samantha pursued things with another group of friends. That left Steve and me time to share meals and weekends together—alone. We spent most Friday nights going out to dinner or watching movies. As friendships dissolved around me, Steve seemed to be the one solid person I could count on. *He makes me laugh, he's friendly and polite. I like being around him.* Steve was ultimately becoming my best friend.

During one semester, my Cross Cultural Communication class required that I attend a variety of evening diversity programs. Steve agreed to go with me. He had more free time now that the basketball season was over. On one particular Friday night, we planned to go out for dinner at Jefferson's and then to an Indian music performance. Fridays left me exhausted. Although it would be a challenging night, I wasn't about to give in and stay home.

"I'll pick you up." Steve's gray Ford F150 pulled up, and after dinner, we headed over to the Performing Arts Center on campus, which meant I would receive some extra credit for my class. I never knew if the extra points would pull me out of a bind, so I looked at them as an insurance policy. Paul Lewiston's legacy, I suppose …

The performance ended at 8:30 P.M.—late by my Friday night standards. *My body is feeling every moment that I lived today.* As we step outside, I could feel the warm May breeze move through my ponytail. I took a few steps on the sidewalk and stopped. I caught my balance, took three more steps and stopped again. Steve was just a single long step ahead of me. I felt my frustration growing—*I would love to be able to walk next to him and not have him wait for me. I can do this.* I started to count my steps in my head, since that usually helped me focus and keep my balance. *One, two, three, four, five, stop. I want to scream, but I will stay positive. We are only two blocks from my apartment. College students walked this path like it was nothing each and every day. Step, step, step, clomp. I wish I had my scooter!*

"Need a hand?" Steve turned to me.

"No, thanks," I smiled, taking another two heavy steps.

Step, step, clomp.

"Are you sure you don't need a hand? I don't mind," Steve assured me.

"No, I'll be fine." I didn't ever take help from people at school. Sure, if I needed help clearing the snow off of my car or carrying in a heavy bag of groceries, I accepted *that* kind of help—only because any girl on campus would.

Steve and I finally reached my apartment. I grasped the metal doorknob and awkwardly lunged forward, bumping into the door. Unsure if I would be able to take another step, I practically fell inside my living room, where I immediately dropped onto the ugly plaid couch near my roommate, Emily. Steve sat on the other sofa in the room, and we visited as we watched television the rest of the evening.

At 11:00 P.M., Steve told me goodbye and I knew that I would see him again soon. I was so thankful to have him as a friend. *There are not too many people who would share that dreadful walk with me, and still stick around for TV.*

* * *

I was down to the final week of my senior year in college. *Four years flew by so quickly. I have accomplished so much! There are many people that didn't think I would be able to do this, myself included. In one week I will be putting on my black robe and walking across a stage to get my diploma that proves I have a BA in organizational communication.* I was so excited!

I wanted to secure As in Communication Studies and Native America History. Professor Wilkinson didn't put a limit on extra credit, so my final weekend was going to be an extra credit marathon. I picked up a half a dozen vintage movies about people of different races. *All I have to do is watch them and type up a one-page analysis for each one in order to get ten points for each.* Steve called and asked if I could get together tonight.

"Sorry. I have to watch all these movies this weekend. I need this A, and the extra credit will guarantee my grade."

He offered to come over and watch some of them with me. "Sounds good. See you soon."

I had the movies all ready to go in my bedroom. This was one of those nights I was thankful I lived in the basement since it was a hot, muggy night. I wore comfortable jean shorts and a T-shirt, and I still kept a fan going in my bedroom to keep the air moving. As soon as I heard a knock on the door, I walked to the living room to let Steve inside. As usual, he looked handsome. Tonight, he was wearing his white T-shirt that said, "Basketball Is Life."

"Do you mind if we watch the movies in my room?" I asked Steve as I lead him down the hall to the bedrooms.

"That's fine," he said, following me.

Steve sat on the middle of the twin bed I had used as a couch for years. I put the Whoopi Goldberg movie in ... *The Long Walk Home.* As soon as I saw the opening credits on the screen, I took a few steps and dropped onto the bed not far from Steve. This was the closest the two of us had ever sat next to one another in the two years that I had known him. Yet, I didn't give it much thought. It was just Steve.

By the time the movie was over, I had jotted down a few notes on a piece of paper as reference for the paper I would write the next day. Steve informed me that he was hungry and I offered to make him chicken Kiev.

He looked slightly surprised as I walked into the kitchen, preheated the oven, and tossed a frozen hunk onto a cookie sheet before putting it into the oven. I set the timer for thirty-five minutes and walked back to my bedroom to place the next movie into the VCR. I sat back in my spot, smiled at Steve, and looked back at the television. Thirty-five minutes later, I went back to the kitchen to retrieve his snack. When I handed it to him, he chuckled and said, "I thought you were making this homemade."

I laughed out loud, "If there is one thing you should know about me, it's that I don't cook."

I sat back down beside him and tried to watch the movie. *I'm not sure what it is, but something seems different tonight. This doesn't feel like a normal night with Steve.* I tried to focus on the movie and continue looking at the screen. As soon as the end credits scrolled up, I popped off of the bed to put the next movie in. But, I realized I needed a walk to the bathroom before I started back on the movie marathon.

As I struggled walking back from the bathroom, I decided to shut the door behind me to prevent noise from my roommates interfering with the next movie. I turned to approach my seat at the bed. I was stunned to see Steve sitting with one arm extended, right where I had been sitting all evening.

I wasn't quite sure what to do. *Do I sit in my same spot and have his arm around me or do I sit on the floor as I have always done in the past?* This had never happened to me before.

I slowly walked to the bed, sat down, scooted myself back onto his arm, in the exact same spot I had been sitting all night. I assumed that if he didn't want his arm around me, he would quickly take it back anyway.

Okay, as long as his arm is around me I cannot possibly concentrate on this movie.

It's been ten minutes and his arm is still around me.

He intentionally placed his arm there so he could be closer to me, right? My mind was racing with ideas, but none of them had anything to do with the movie.

My roommate Emily knocked on the door.

"Come in," I said.

"You have a phone call … " Emily started to say, but clearly the shock of seeing Steve and me cuddled together in front of a movie stopped her thought. She simply grinned and handed me the phone, before turning, walking away, and closing the door behind her.

The phone call was a classmate wondering about the extra credit option. "Yep—just a one-pager for each movie you watch."

Another movie was half over, but this time I had no idea what it was about. All I could think of was how I had somehow wound up snuggled up with my good friend Steve—and it felt perfect!

"My arm is starting to fall asleep."

"Oh, sorry." I leaned forward so he could move and get some life back into his limb. Stretching onto his side, I somehow had fallen over with him. I tried to picture this in my mind, since I wasn't paying attention to the movie anyway—*we're lying together on my bed watching … or trying to watch … or pretending to watch, a movie that I need to write a paper on tomorrow.*

My head rested against his chest. I looked up at him and I couldn't seem to look away. We stared intently into one another's eyes for several moments. *Is he going to kiss me? Why won't he kiss me? He really should kiss me. Does he want to kiss me? He better kiss me! Maybe he doesn't want to kiss me. Maybe he's not sure if he should kiss me. Do I need to kiss him? Does he want me to kiss him? But I can't risk him rejecting me.*

I leaned toward his face and gently kissed his right eye. *God, why did I kiss his eye! This is worse than Jennifer Grey telling Patrick Swayze she carried a watermelon in the movie* Dirty Dancing. *I should have gone for it and just kissed him!*

But then Steve turned his head and kissed me on the mouth,

right as it should have been from the start. His mouth was perfect. His kisses were soft and slow. *He can kiss me for a really long time. I don't want him to stop.* He must have felt the same way, because the kiss lasted for nearly an hour.

When we stopped kissing, I turned to the clock and saw that it was after one in the morning. It was time for Steve to go home, so I walked him to the door that led outside. He found his shoes where he had left them at my front door. He put them on while I opened the door, and we said goodnight to one another. He leaned down and kissed me again before turning and heading for home. I closed the door, shook my head, and smiled in disbelief as I walked to my bedroom for a night of pretend sleep.

Georgia on My Mind

STEVE AND I SPENT EVERY FREE MOMENT TOGETHER OVER the next week. We hung out at the lake, ate at either his place or my place for dinner, and essentially held hands and/or kissed as often as possible. *I'm twenty-one years old and I'm just realizing for the first time what it means to have a boyfriend.*

Only two days remained before Steve had to leave for the summer. He couldn't stay for my graduation because his best friend was getting married the same day and Steve was in the wedding. Although he asked me to attend the wedding with him, I chose to walk for my graduation ... such a milestone for me and my family. I began to wonder, *What will happen to us now that Steve is leaving for the summer and I am going home to decide on my next step after graduation? I'm done with my degree, but Steve will return in the fall to finish his ... and I won't be here. Will this relationship just fizzle out? What does he think of "us"?* He was coming over that evening, so I planned to find the courage to ask him what he thought of our future ... if anything.

My stomach was a tangle of knots as I waited for Steve in my apartment that night. I was excited to be with him, yet nervous to find out if he viewed me as his girlfriend ... *or am I just some girl that he's been making out with the past week?* He didn't seem like that kind of guy. My *friend* Steve never talked about girls before I became more than a friend to him.

Later in the evening, Steve and I were cuddled up on my bed watching another movie that neither one of us really cared to see.

Our time together was limited. He leaned in, and brushed his lips against mine in a sweet kiss that quickly turned passionate. *When I'm in his arms, nothing else matters.* When he pulled away, I looked up into his big brown eyes and neither one of us spoke for a moment. I broke the silence.

"What are we?" I said with concerned eyes. The thought of not seeing him once I moved back home made my heart sink. *I'm not sure what I'll do without him.* I thought about telling him this, but Steve spoke before I could.

Assuring me that we were a couple, Steve looked directly at me and said, "You're my girlfriend." I smiled, and the tangled knots in my stomach unraveled and dissolved as I grew in confidence that we would not be giving each other up.

The next few months found us taking turns—driving nearly three hours each way to be together on the weekends. I watched the clock every night, waiting for the synchronized time we had set for an hour-long talk on the phone. I couldn't wait until he'd break into the country song "Drink, Swear, Steal and Lie." Steve's voice was wonderful, and this gave me a moment to acknowledge that I had fallen in love—I couldn't imagine living my life without him.

I had secured an amazing internship for the summer. My weekdays were filled with teaching workshops for welfare participants at the Minnesota Workforce Center in Blaine. I lucked out with a manageable walk from the parking space marked Handicapped, to a rather small building. My energy level getting to work was spared. Thus, I had endurance to last a full shift. I also found motivation in the thought that perhaps I helped some of the welfare participants in a subtler way. I secretly hoped that, after watching me struggle physically to do my job, they found returning to the workforce less daunting. This possibility made my service to them even more rewarding. I was motivated by the hope that my difficulty around the classroom or computer room inspired others to get back to a more self-sufficient life.

My internship was nearing its end. I was fortunate to find a job with HIRED in Brooklyn Center as an employment counselor,

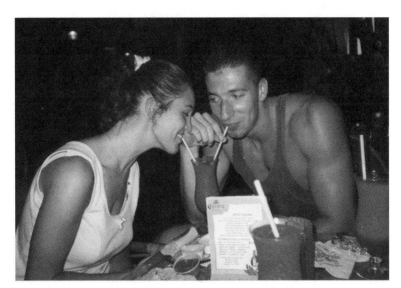

Jean and Steve in Fort Lauderdale, Florida

to help clients find work, and in time, no longer need public assistance. Again, I felt such reward in knowing that despite my disability, I worked in a helping profession—I had skills to contribute to the lives of so many able-bodied people. This motivated me to do the best job I could ... yet change for Steve and me was inevitable. I feared my future happiness since a fulfilling career was not the only thing I wanted anymore.

Steve would be starting school soon and the basketball season would be in full swing. *We won't be spending every weekend together.* The thought of Steve spending his weekends at out-of-town games made my heart fall.

My job at HIRED became more demanding as I had a caseload of nearly ninety welfare participants by fall. My job to help them find jobs became stressful. It was apparent to me that only one person on my caseload truly wanted to get off of the benefits provided by MFIP, Minnesota Family Investment Program. At times, I felt as if I was a full-time babysitter rather than an employment counselor.

My own employment reviews were based on how many of my clients received jobs while on my watch. The fact was, the majority of those with whom I worked didn't want employment. I sanctioned their checks, which meant a substantial financial reduction, but they still didn't show up for workshops that would help them prepare for interviews or new skills if hired.

The stress began to build and affect my sleep in the worst way. As it always did, my lack of sleep impacted my mobility. I was exhausted when I went to bed and usually woke up at 4:00 A.M., worried about my clients. Would they turn in their paperwork, due at the beginning of the week, or go to their job interviews that I had arranged? The year ticked along, and so did the strain. The only thing that kept me going were my supportive co-workers—and knowing that I would see Steve whenever possible.

On May 13, I arrived at work to see a dozen red roses sitting on my desk with a note from Steve. It was our one-year anniversary. I leaned over to smell the soft floral scent and I wished I could hop in my car to drive to Winona. Unfortunately, this whim to see him would have to wait a few days. I'd have to settle for a phone call until the weekend.

* * *

Another hot summer made me thankful for air conditioning. Without it, my lack of sleep would have jeopardized my health even more, and my walking would have worsened. *I just wish that Steve could come this weekend. There's no one else that I would rather spend my birthday with.* But I knew that Steve's summer work schedule made it impossible for him to visit—even when the occasion was my twenty-third birthday.

That summer, Steve called me nightly around 9:30 when he was on his break at Pella Windows in Iowa, five hours away. Even though I needed my sleep, I couldn't pass up the opportunity to hear his voice for those fifteen minutes every day.

This time, he reminded me, "I can't come this weekend. I'm sorry it won't work out."

"I know. I understand. It's just too much driving," I replied, although it made me so sad to think we wouldn't be together on my birthday. "I understand it, but that doesn't make it any easier."

It was time for Steve to get back to work.

"I gotta go, I love you," he said softly into the phone.

"I love you too, Steve. Goodnight." Neither of us hung up the phone. The silence was deafening, yet I sat there and listened to silence for another ten seconds.

"We'd better go. I love you."

"I love you too."

"Goodnight," I said, finally hanging up so I didn't have to endure the silence any more.

On Friday, I awoke at 5:00 A.M. to the sound of rain. *I've never heard rain like this before. It almost sounds like hail.* Half asleep, I tried to figure it out. *Why is there only one pebble of hail hitting my window each time—and at twenty-second intervals? Oh, my gosh! It's not raining! And that's not hail!*

I jumped out of my bed and peeked through the blinds covering my bedroom window. I looked down to see Steve looking back at me. *He's so beautiful!* I turned away from my window and trudged down the flight of stairs that led to my front door. I scrambled to unlock the door to greet Steve with a huge, tight hug.

"I've never seen you move so fast," he teased.

"You came for my birthday." Johnny Depp would not have played this part any better.

I screamed and hugged him again as I released all of my excitement. *This may be the happiest moment of my life. I'm living in a romantic film … stuff like this only happens in the movies, right?*

"I have to go to bed," Steve stated, exhaustion in his voice. After working all evening, then driving through the night, who could blame him? But he was here! And that was what mattered.

I took him down to the basement, where he slept for every visit to my parents' home. He took a box out of his bag and handed it to me. "Here, you can have your birthday gift now."

I slowly took it from his hands. *You being here was the only gift I really wanted.* But I opened the wooden box to find a beautiful watch. He helped me put it on and then stated in a lifeless voice, "I really need to sleep."

I hugged him, went back to my room, and collapsed on my twin bed. *There's no way I'll be able to go back to sleep after this excitement.* I got dressed and went to work. *All I have to do is get through today and the weekend will be spent with my Steve.*

Summer was nearing the end and, along with it, Steve's internship. He called me one afternoon to inform me that he had been offered a job in Macon, Georgia. The details of the job offer helped me see what a great opportunity this was, but I couldn't stop the sickness in my stomach. I played with the white phone cord as he told me how much he really wanted this job.

"I want you to come with me," he said with confidence.

I wasn't sure what to think, but I knew that I couldn't move with him to another side of the country if we were not married. "I'm not going to follow you around the country like a puppy dog," I said with sternness in my voice. *I'm not going to let him have his cake and eat it too.* This cliché, and so many about a guy who "promised" marriage, but showed no sign of a plan, came racing into my mind. Too many movie scenes warned me to get a true commitment, or I would be the sad, disabled girl who returned home to her parents, single, alone, and unloved.

But Steve was not an actor ... I listened to his plans, and let my guard down long enough to imagine us living together in Georgia. "I promise—we'll get engaged after we move. I just don't want this move to be the reason I am proposing."

I understood his point, but I just couldn't help wondering, *If he had to, would he go without me?*

"At least come with me to see if this is a place where you could live."

I agreed. I would go with him for a visit.

The following weeks, every conversation ended with us fighting and me in tears. *I don't want to move to Georgia with a boyfriend. How stupid does that look?* I wasn't sure if our relationship could handle this test. *God, I need your guidance more than ever! Do I stay or do I go with the love of my life?*

Then the day came—Steve and I prepared to pull out of my driveway in my grey Mercury Sable, headed toward the airport. I looked out the passenger window to watch my dad mount his John Deere riding lawnmower. The grass was lush and green. Like every summer, Dad's hard work had paid off again. With the car still in park, Steve jerked the car door open.

"I'll be right back," Steve said, jumping out of the car. He briskly walked over to my dad. They talked for just over a minute. I actually timed them. *What is going on?* With both of their backs to me, I couldn't even attempt to lip read. As Steve turned away from my dad, I watched as he walked toward me, opened the car door, and hopped back into the driver's seat. This memory is still vivid to me. I was so concerned and curious, yet it never dawned on me that Steve was asking for my dad's permission to marry me.

"What was that all about?"

"I was just telling him when I thought we'd be back."

If I wasn't so stressed out about my future, I think I would have pressed for more information. I was just too tired to care at that moment.

Our flight to Atlanta was on time. You'd think we'd have had plenty to discuss with all that was happening, but our ability to hold a conversation seemed broken. My stress level caused my body to disengage from my brain. My life felt as if it were hanging in the hands of Steve Abbott. Yet I knew deep down inside that the decision was ultimately mine.

We spent the next two days discovering the lush green city of Macon, finding it to be a manageable place, with apartments we could afford. I really liked the one-bedroom off Interstate 175. It looked brand new, and listed at less than $600 a month. You couldn't live in an ice shack for that price back in Minnesota. The agent looked at us, "So, do you want to sign the lease?"

Steve turned to me. I looked into his big, brown, hopeful eyes. *How could I possibly leave him?*

"Let's do it," I said, smiling up at him.

We continued our vacation even after our plane brought us back to the Midwest. Steve had booked a room at The Carriage House Bed and Breakfast in Winona. We had stayed there about a year ago when we first started dating. We walked into the small entry and put some snack-sized chocolate bars into our pockets before we went to our room. We were both exhausted from the past two days and the stress from imagining such a big move. We fell asleep in each other's arms ... a sign that I was finally comfortable with all this change in my life.

At 5:00 A.M., Steve gently pushed on my shoulder. "Let's watch the sunrise up at Garvin Heights."

I barely opened my eyes. "I need to sleep."

"Come on, it'll be fun." Steve nudged me again.

I agreed and reluctantly got out of bed. I grabbed my Minneapolis phone book out of my suitcase for my morning stretches.

"Do that when we get back. We don't want to miss the sunrise," Steve pushed.

I sighed in irritation, but put my sneakers on anyway.

* * *

After driving to the highest point, we parked, and walked hand-in-hand up the slight paved incline to reach the overlook of Garvin Heights. I felt it in my calves that I had skipped my morning stretch routine. *We're late.* The sun stretched out over the city's horizon. Apparently Steve was not the only one with the romantic idea of spying on the first light of day. A dozen people dotted the bluff-top.

We sat in a quiet spot and scanned the city below us. *Winona will forever be the place where this wonderful man and I were brought together.* From this distance, the city looked deserted. We sat quietly together and enjoyed the view. Slowly, the other viewers got into their cars and left the overlook.

"Ready to go?" I said, balancing to push myself up to a standing position. As I began moving in the direction of my car, Steve stopped me suddenly.

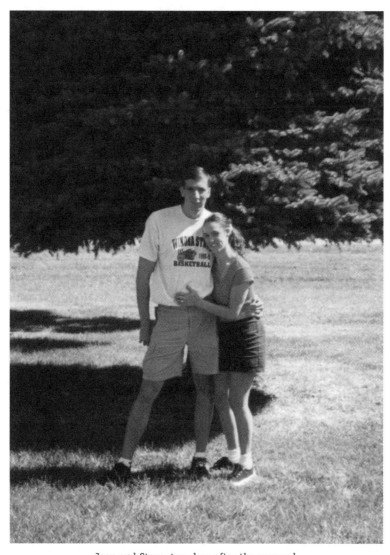

Jean and Steve, two days after the proposal

"Wait," he said. I turned around to face him. His right hand was fumbling around in the pocket of his khaki shorts. I stared at his movement and saw a slight sparkle peeking out from the pocket of his shorts.

"Shut up!" I said as soon as I realized it was a diamond causing that sparkle.

Steve took a few short steps in my direction and got down on one knee, "Will you marry me?"

Shocked, not by his question, but by the very fact that I so cluelessly did not see this coming, I shouted, "Yes!" I wrapped my arms around him and hugged him as tightly as I could.

When he pulled away, he took the solitaire ring and tried to place it on my finger.

It was clearly too small, but before a glimmer of disappointment could touch this moment, Steve placed the ring on my pinkie.

Frankly, I didn't care where he put the ring. I just wanted to be his wife.

Disabled in the
Grown-Up World

IN LESS THAN THREE WEEKS, WITH THE HELP OF MY MOM, we booked the church, reception venue, photographer, flowers, and ordered the cake. *Georgia, here I come.*

From wedding plans to the big move, Mom and I were really proud of ourselves for making the trip to Macon, Georgia, in two short days—with a little help from MapQuest. We pulled into my new apartment and were stunned to see my dad's suburban, and the trailer with all of my belongings, in the parking spot next to us.

"How did they make it here before us?" I shrieked, looking at my mom in disbelief.

My dad and Tom had left a whole day later than us. Refusing to unload until we got the full story, the guys finally admitted, "We never stopped to sleep."

"No hotel?" I asked in disbelief.

"No hotel," Dad stated with a prideful grin. "We were wide awake, so we thought, why not drive through the night?"

Steve greeted everyone, then helped my family unload my brown flowered couches—I still remember the print, with birds seemingly camouflaged throughout the fabric. This may not have been my first choice for furniture, but when my parents offered items from their formal living room, I couldn't say no. Having furniture handed to us would be a big savings for Steve and me.

We spent the afternoon together—working, unloading, arranging my new home. I was fully aware of the fact that my family would be leaving soon. *This isn't supposed to be sad. Why am I so sad? I've lived away from my parents and my brothers before. Why does this have to feel so different? So final?*

I gave each a hug goodbye. The three of them jumped into the Suburban, put the windows down, and happily waved to me. My stomach began to flutter as I held onto Steve's side. I returned their love with a wave and a smile to hide my tears. *In twenty-three years of life, I've never been this far away from family. I didn't see this coming, but this is harder than leaving them for college.*

After I watched the bumper of the black vehicle drive out of sight, I looked up at Steve and smiled. *A very bittersweet moment. I have the man that I dreamed of, but never thought possible, yet my family will be a two-day drive away.* Steve and I turned to enter our one-bedroom apartment. *It will all be okay. And I will become a stronger, more independent person because of this.* My pep talks with God would continue nonstop throughout the next few weeks.

The job search provided a welcomed distraction from homesickness. After a month of looking and a handful of interviews, I accepted a position at a small employment agency called Walter's Workforce. I was relieved that I didn't have to focus on welfare recipients this time. My life would no longer be dependent upon what others did—or *didn't* do—with their lives. The Walter's Workforce office had only four employees: Walter, his daughter Audrey, Julie, and me. Walter, an overweight, fifty-something, gray-haired grandpa seemed to be procrastinating my training. I would have to help out in the office until there was time to train me for the actual position I filled. I explained to Steve, "He's informed me that they are going to wait to train me. He said that he needs to get the other girl trained first."

As I started working in the small office, I felt unsure about my duties. For days, I helped fill temporary positions, which was primarily the task of assisting those who were looking for temp work through our agency. I was used to treating every candidate the same. Sure, I had been frustrated at my old job in Minnesota when clients skipped the steps needed to find the next job. But I acted professionally. I treated each client with respect, even when I had to deliver the consequences of reduced benefits. But now, as a resident of Georgia, I was confronted with blatant racism for the first time in my life. Walter and his daughter both instructed me in the procedures of differentiating between white and black applicants for temp positions. I had been explicitly told that with black applicants, I needed to put a distinct mark at the top left hand corner of their note cards.

"Sometimes, we need to make sure we send a white person to a job," or "we like to try and fill the position with a white person if we can." Walter's daughter made these remarks as if this was simply a reminder of normal procedure. *Wow, they don't even try to cover up what they are doing.* They showed clear favoritism toward one race, and they made no secret about it.

The first time I heard this directive from Audrey, I couldn't help but wonder if she was serious. I paged through all the clients' paperwork and saw that indeed several of the pages had a *W* at the top. *I can't do this. It's just not right.* As I helped a variety of candidates fill out their paperwork, I deliberately ignored the office policy, and left the racial markings off the tops of the cards.

I was grateful for the small office. Our front door chimes sounded when someone entered—my cue to start making my way to the counter. I couldn't exactly sprint to someone's aid, but the clients didn't seem to mind waiting. They usually smiled at me as I struggled my way up front. Julie had told me that all the phone calls needed to be answered on the first ring, but my arms just couldn't work that fast. I typically grabbed the receiver by the third ring.

Two months into my job, I still hadn't officially been trained. Yet, the clients seemed to like me, and I had filled many positions before their deadlines. Walter and his daughter always greeted me with a smile and asked how things were going. I had told them all about growing up disabled, and they seem to appreciate my hard work to accomplish what I had so far in life. At least that's what I thought.

"Jean, can you come into my office?" Walter said at the end of one workweek.

"Sure," I said, slowly walking back to his office.

I wasn't sure what he had to say, but his daughter joined us and closed the door.

"Jean, we need to cut your pay," Walter said, his eyes on the floor ahead of him.

I couldn't imagine why he was saying this. However, just two weeks prior to this moment, I had asked Walter if there was a way for me to get a pay increase or health insurance. I was making far less than I did in Minnesota. I knew it was a small company, but when I asked for this increase, he simply said that now was not the time. He didn't make any mention of cutting my pay.

Walter proceeded to tell me that they were not getting what they needed out of me on a daily basis. "You don't get to the counter fast enough, and you never answer the phone on the first ring," Walter explained.

As he filled me in on all of my faults, I stopped listening to his justification for this cut. All my focus went toward preventing my tears from falling from my stunned eyes.

"Don't get us wrong," his daughter added. "This has nothing to do with your disability."

Walter informed me that I could take the weekend to think about whether I would return to work after a pay cut. "We understand if you want to resign."

As I squeaked out an "okay," I slowly got up from the chair, grabbed my car keys from my desk, and walked out into the heat of the Georgia sun. I was not sure how this had happened. *My whole life, I have been told what a hard worker I am ... and how I don't let my disability interfere with my work. Yes, I needed some accommodations, but I never thought this would cost me my job. I thought people admired my will to work.*

My slightly slower pace seemed to help everyone take a patient breath and appreciate what skills they had to bring to the dignity of work. I thought I had been an inspiration, not a hindrance. Had I been fooling myself?

I opened the door to the apartment. Steve greeted me with a smile, but stood up from the couch, sensing something was wrong.

As soon as our eyes met, my tears began falling like a waterfall after a flood.

The concern on Steve's face became graver when I started to hyperventilate.

"What's wrong?"

My crying was so out of control that I couldn't talk. Somehow, between gasps, I found the words.

"They're cutting my pay!" I cried out in a loud wheeze for breath.

"What?" Steve said, walking towards me. "Tell me what happened."

"I can't!" I ran to the bathroom and closed the door.

All of the stress caused my stomach to cramp up. I struggled to get my pants down just as the diarrhea hit. As I sat on the toilet crying like I did when my cat died ten years ago, I felt like I would vomit. Steve waited patiently on the other side of the door—I'm not sure for how long. But finally, I walked out of the bathroom and sat down next to him to pour out the information I was told less than an hour ago.

"They said it had nothing to do with my disability," I said, throwing my head forward and drowning my face in my hands. "What am I going to do?"

"You're quitting. You don't need to go back there," Steve said, putting his arm around me.

"I need to work," I insisted.

"Not there," Steve said.

Then, after a moment, "Maybe we should move back."

I could tell that he felt responsible.

"No," I whispered. "That's not going to make me feel better about this." *We can't move back. We came here for your career. I can't be the reason.*

Steve sat with me while I cried off and on for the next hour. After a long talk, we decided that I would not return to work at Walter's Workforce, and that I would find another job—a better one. Over the weekend, Steve sat with me as I called and left a voicemail on Walter's phone: "I won't be returning to work."

I was finding that life in Georgia was not the same as life in Minnesota. *People don't seem to be as accepting of my disability, but I will not let it stop me from getting a job.* Unlike many women my age in Georgia, I had a degree—and I intended to use it.

The following Monday, I made a phone call to the Department of Rehabilitation and told them that I needed their assistance in finding a job. Two days later, I met with Mr. King, who helped me with many contacts in the Macon area. Less than three weeks later, I was hired as a service representative for the Social Security Administration. There was a reason why my job at Walter's Workforce didn't work out—I was meant to be a government employee. The annual salary was $10,000 more than Walter's Workforce. Plus, I had excellent health insurance, and I was quite confident that they weren't going to discriminate against me because of my disability.

There seemed to be another reason why my job at Walter's Workforce did not work out. We knew that what Walter and his daughter did to me was not only wrong, but illegal, so we decided to contact an attorney. If we had any chance at a lawsuit against them, it wouldn't be about money. It would be about putting a stop to this with any future employees.

I spoke with an attorney over the phone and he sent me paperwork to fill out with the Equal Employment Opportunity Commission. As soon as the EEOC responded back, the attorney called me into his office. Steve and I drove there, and as the attorney shook my hand, he stated, "You definitely have a case."

He explained, "Your boss at Walter's Workforce completed his portion of the EEOC paperwork and claimed that he and his staff never knew you were disabled."

"What? That's absurd. I shared with him—and his daughter—so many things about growing up with a disability. I thought they were impressed with me at the time. I thought they admired me for all of my hard work to be independent. Pretty naïve on my part … but they're lying when they say they didn't know."

He informed me that any judge or jury would see I was disabled pretty quickly. "I saw how your arm appeared spastic as we shook hands. And if those in the courtroom saw you walk, they would know that Walter was lying about everything."

"Clearly, the man lied in his EEOC paperwork." But then the attorney said something so unexpected to us. "But, I'll be honest, filing a claim would not be worth your time." Our surprised faces prompted him to share more—to justify why an open-and-shut case should not be pursued. "You said yourself, you've got a much better job now," he said, leaning back in his chair. "And it only took you a few weeks to find it. You were wise to use the Department of Rehabilitation's help."

I looked at Steve. Both of us seemed speechless.

"If you file a suit, it will tie you and Steve down for three years and lead to very little compensation."

"But, I don't want them to do this to someone else," I finally retorted.

"Of course not. And now that a file has been completed with the EEOC, I don't think Walter and his staff will do this again. And if they do, there's already plenty on their record." The attorney sounded so sure that dropping the suit was the best thing to do.

Steve and I followed the attorney's advice. We let it go. Our jobs and wedding plans took precedence over a potentially long legal battle. I only hoped that calling Walter out on his discriminatory ways was enough to keep him from treating other employees unfairly.

Eight months later, Steve and I were back in Minnesota ... not to live, but to get married. Thanks to my family, all of the wedding preparations were completed. We decided on a small wedding party, so I asked Amy Stockamp to be my maid of honor, and Steve's sister to be my bridesmaid. I wanted to have other friends as well, but felt that family was important at this event. It would be so hard to decide on just one friend, anyway—unless I wanted the wedding party to be half the guest list!

Steve asked his brother to be his best man, his friend Allen to be his groomsman, and my brothers to be ushers. Because I wanted a wedding that was simple yet elegant, I wanted my flowers to be the same way. They looked perfect—as if I had just picked them from the wild that morning. Plus, I knew they had to be lightweight. Most of our pictures were taken before the wedding—early enough so I wouldn't look worn out. During the large group photo, I was starting to lean forward, but my dress camouflaged this pretty well. Steve held me up as the photographer worked his magic. Luckily for me, this was the best day physically I had ever had, so I was able to stand taller and straighter than normal. I now know that God was truly by my side that day. Things couldn't have been more perfect.

Our reception, set for Majestic Oaks Golf Club, included a prime rib buffet and a surprise ice sculpture of lovebirds kissing—one of my parents' gifts. Periwinkle wildflowers that matched my bridesmaids' dresses adorned the sculpture and tables. Our wedding was at 11:00 A.M. and our reception followed right after. The dance started around three and was done by seven—not your typical wedding day schedule. But we knew an early wedding, if I were to endure the rigor of a reception and dance, would be the only way for me to enjoy the day. I think Steve knew early on the truth behind the old cliché, "happy wife, happy life." Or, in my case, comfortable, well-rested wife meant no worries for this once-in-a-lifetime event!

Our rehearsal day meant Steve would spend the afternoon with his dad, sister, and brother, and I would spend the day with my folks. Mom and I were reviewing a few details when the phone interrupted our small talk. She ran upstairs to pick up, then called, "Jean, it's for you."

I made my way up the flight of stairs to what used to be my bedroom. It was now decorated in an angel theme. I sat on the white chair, next to my old purple and white phone—a gift when I turned fifteen.

I picked the receiver up off the glass tabletop. "Hello," I said.

"Hello, Miss Jean." I heard the unmistakable voice on the other line. Short Steve. *What a surprise*, I thought to myself.

"I just called to congratulate you on your wedding tomorrow," I heard him say.

I wasn't sure what to think. *Was he about to try to get me back?*

"Thanks," I said. "It's too bad that it never worked out between us."

I'll never know why I said that. I definitely didn't mean it. I guess I just didn't know how to respond to the situation. The phone call didn't last much longer. In fact, I think it was the shortest phone call I had ever shared with him. We said goodbye and I hung up the phone without an ounce of hesitation.

Our rehearsal was flawless. I could not have asked for it to be any more special, including our dinner at the Season's Restaurant. As I got into my parents' car, Steve kissed me goodbye.

"I'll see you at the altar at 11:00 A.M.," I smiled at him.

After Steve carefully closed my car door, Dad drove us home. *The next time I see Steve we'll be ready to say our vows.* To this day, I still can't find words to describe the excitement and joy of that evening … the anticipation of something I couldn't fathom even two years ago.

We arrived home about 9:30 P.M., my bedtime. I set the alarm for 6:30 A.M. and took the prescribed sleeping pill that I had been taking for over a year. I also swallowed the blue Tylenol PM that the neurologist said would be okay to add as extra insurance that I would get solid sleep. As I looked at my reflection in the bedroom mirror, I prayed. *God, please help me get a good night's sleep. Tomorrow is the most important day of my life and more than anything I want to enjoy every moment of it. I want to be that beautiful, confident bride who can walk down the isle toward her groom. I want to stand with ease as I say "I do." And I desperately want to have that first dance with Steve. Please, let me have this day one day where I can feel stronger than ever before.*

At 6:30 A.M., the pink clock radio played its peppy song. I quickly got out of my bed to do a little victory dance, the best I could. *I just had the best night of sleep ever! Thank you, God, for answering my prayers!* I looked into the little white mirror and smiled at the girl looking back at me. I couldn't help but squeal.

"I'm getting married today!"

I put on a pair of jean shorts, the corset bra that I would wear under my wedding gown, and one of my mom's button-down plaid sleeveless shirts. I ran down the stairs just as I had so many Christmases past. Only today would be better than Christmas! I already discovered my present—the gift of sleep. I downed a glass of milk along with a slice of my mom's homemade banana bread. *We are off to get our hair done.*

My mom drove us to Designers on 18, and not long after we arrived, Amy and Jenny were sitting in the salon chairs next to me. I handed over the simple yet elegant veil to the stylist. "Mom and I found this at David's Bridal nine months ago," I explained. "I just want a simple bun." My stylist did a fantastic job getting my hair tucked into a classic bun, and then secured the two-foot veil to it. Little wisps of leftover hair were curled with an iron to add the finishing touches. She turned me to face the mirror and I saw exactly what I wanted to see: simplicity. *I want to look special, but not like a stranger.*

My mom's hair was finished shortly after mine, so she drove me to the church. In the parking lot, I turned to her with my plea, "Can you go in and make sure Steve won't see me get out of the car?"

Given a new mission, Mom walked into the church and then back to the beige Buick. She gave me the okay signal and together we marched into the church. We headed down the short hallway to the bridal room on the left. The gold carpeting reminded us that St. Patrick's Church was built the year I was born. I was one of the last babies to be baptized in the old church before this one was built in 1976. Now, here I was in 2000, as one of the last brides to walk down the aisle. A bigger St. Patrick's was already under construction to accommodate many new parishioners. With a little over one hundred guests coming, the "old church" was a perfect setting.

My sisters-in-law, both personal attendants, met us in the bridal room with their two beautiful daughters. Cathy and Michelle had their kids sitting quietly in their strollers. Although these little girls are cousins, you would never guess it. Mikaela has dark olive skin, with big chocolate brown eyes and brunette hair that has been kissed by the Minnesota summer sun. While Sophia, just one year younger, has the skin of Snow White, white-blonde hair that stands straight up in her little ponytail, and blue-gray eyes that remind me so much of my Grandma Sharon.

"I brought makeup," Cathy announced as she dug into her bag.

I hadn't even thought about makeup, I admitted only to myself. Ten minutes later, Cathy held up a mirror to reveal the outcome of her artistry. The reflection smiled back at me. The makeup matched the hair ... simple yet elegant. *Cathy knows me well.*

"Are you thirsty?" Cathy placed a big white bedsheet over my dress. She handed me a Styrofoam cup with a little red straw for my mouth. I sipped the water and looked around at all the women present to share this day with me. Just then Jenny, Steve's sister, walked in.

"Have you seen Steve this morning?" I asked, leaning forward. "How is he doing?"

"He seems nervous," she said nonchalantly.

Part of me wished I could see Steve—I could help calm his nerves before the big event. I wanted him to have as much fun with the preliminary festivities as I was having. But we'd made a pact not to see each other until the ceremony started.

The wedding director brought our attention back to the reason we were here. She informed those in the bridal room, "It's just about time," which drew my mind back to all of the details of the ceremony. The organist's opening notes from our chosen song, "Friends are Friends Forever," made the vocalist seem angelic. I was remarkably calm, but a little wishful that I was hiding out in the crowd to hear and see it all unfold. Only a few short years ago, I truly believed this day would never happen—that I would never share my life with someone—especially a person as wonderful as Steve.

We shuffled to the back of the church as the song neared its end. *I am getting married.* Thinking back now, I know it was divine intervention. I walked with such ease—this couldn't simply be chalked up to a good night's sleep. God can take all the credit for this.

The wedding party lined up with Steve at the front of the line. "Don't let him turn around and see me," I had instructed his best friend.

The music began once again, and the butterflies in my stomach instantly morphed into bats. With my mom on my left and my dad on my right, I linked my arms in theirs as we prepared to walk down the aisle. I spotted all my friends and family smiling back at me from their pews. Halfway down the aisle I realized I hadn't even looked at Steve. *Where is he?* He quickly drew my attention to the front of the church.

Steve stood with his broad shoulders squared, looking muscular and proud in his sophisticated black tux. His eyes looked at me very

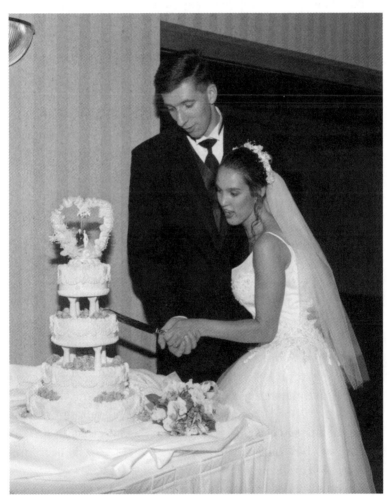

Jean and Steve on their wedding day, July 29, 2000

159

intently, but his smile was welcoming. As I got closer, I thought I saw a hint of a tear in his lovely brown eyes. *This is definitely the man I have waited my whole life for.*

My parents and I reached our final destination. I turned to my father and kissed his tanned cheek. "I love you," I whispered near his ear. *When was the last time I said that to him? It has been a really long time. I bet I was only seven or so.* Those words had gone unspoken, but we both knew that we would do anything for one another. I turned to my mom and hugged her while trying not to crush her pretty corsage. "I love you,"—whispered simultaneously.

I turned to face Steve to take a final step forward. I reached out for his hand. *I need him to help stop the shaking.* Hardly visible, my wildflower bouquet was definitely moving. Steve instinctively linked his hands with mine and tightened his grip around my bouquet stem. His gentle grasp was all I needed. *My doctor has made me better.* The shaking stopped and I could continue on with the ceremony.

We had altered the traditional Catholic wedding mass slightly— accommodations for a bride trying to avoid public displays of spasticity. For instance, the Unity Candle lighting—usually an extra trip up the steps to the altar—could be efficiently performed when we were already standing near the candle. We wanted a fluid, efficient mass with minimal moves for me. We choreographed this just right, and I don't think one person commented or asked, "Why the changes?"

The deacon could have said anything that day. *I hope there isn't a test later. I haven't heard a word so far.* All of my focus was on Steve directly next to me. *He is my everything. Our vows are not cliché—I know that he'll be there during the good times and the bad. How can I be so lucky that God put this man into my life? He can handle my disability. He knows it's just one little part of me. It will not define me.* I know that the deacon touched on these same thoughts, but so far, I had only heard my inner version of them.

Steve and I stood very close while the deacon led us through our vows. *Now* I was paying attention—I had never been so aware of words coming from my mouth before. *Yes, I will honor you. Of course, I will love you all the days of my life. I would never consider disobeying you. You are the love of my life.*

The deacon whispered for the two of us to turn around. He announced us to a church full of loving, caring friends and family: "I now introduce you to Mr. and Mrs. Stephen Abbott!"

It's legit! We are married. I looked at Steve and expected him to lower for a kiss. It was obvious that he wasn't going to until he got permission from the deacon.

"You can kiss me now," I said to him like a little girl on the playground waiting for that first innocent kiss. He didn't move.

"You can kiss me," I whisper again.

Finally, Steve leaned down and brushed his lips against mine ever so lightly for the most appropriate church kiss. I looked out at my friends and they all began to clap. We walked slowly out of the church hand in hand.

I had visualized this final walk for nine months, ever since Steve proposed. I saw Steve scooping me up in his arms, and charging out of the church ... not to be romantic, but to simplify the last part of the ceremonial walk down the aisle. I would be trudging along, dragging my legs—slowing down the celebration. Steve would know what to do—he always did.

Yet, quite the contrary happened. I glided so gracefully. God surely listened to my prayers. No need to scoop Jean up. The potential to trip or fall left all consciousness ... perhaps a glimmer of what was ahead in my life. Yet, I was too ecstatic to even notice, or to imagine life without my walking worries.

None of this mattered as we lined up to hug everyone who came to share in this special day. Mrs. Stephen Abbott had guests to greet.

A Working Mom-To-Be

MY HOLLYWOOD DREAM CAME TRUE! SURE, JOHNNY DEPP was not listed in my wedding program, and our photographer, though amazing, never won an Oscar. I still feel as if I lived the Big Screen for one day in my life. Especially when I discovered my dad had asked the DJ to announce, "The bride and groom are leaving … let's give them a big round of applause!" By the time my brother Tom pulled up our car, everyone had followed us into the parking lot, cheering and whistling. Steve opened the car door for me, and as we pulled away from the crowd, I smiled with the satisfaction that comes from experiencing the perfect wedding day.

We had ten summer days to make a honeymoon drive around Lake Superior. With plenty of stops for hiking and sightseeing, especially along the North Shore, I'm sure people thought we were crazy for wanting to take the rugged paths around Two Harbors, Gooseberry Falls, Thunder Bay, and other remote stops. I can't tell you how many times Steve said, "Here we go—piggyback ride—hop on." He carried me down rocks, reassured me at scary, steep turns, and helped me see vistas I thought impossible. We would never have had the views of the lake and the incredible scenery if Steve hadn't been willing—and strong enough—to carry me. I'm sure the ferry rides at Munising and Sault Ste. Marie brought relief for Steve, but he never complained that his disabled wife hindered our trip. Ten years later, his anniversary gift to me brought us back to the North Shore to retrace our steps after my new diagnosis—where

Steve again guided me, although not as my packhorse. But that's for a later chapter. For now, we toured the scenic North Shore as a newlywed couple with some unusual challenges and a vacationing spirit.

We timed the return from our trip to coincide with Lonnie's wedding in Minnesota. Another happy event kept us away from reality just a little longer. Yet, how could we get Georgia off our minds with jobs and married life waiting for us?

Once back in Georgia, Steve and I became workaholics. I worked first shift. He worked second shift. He worked Saturdays. So, I began working Saturdays too. We made up our minds to build a home—to have something to show for those monthly housing payments. But overachievers that we were, we probably didn't do any better than break even when we sold that home to move back to Minnesota. We tried our best to assimilate as Georgia residents, from October 1999 to May 2002. But for all the nice people who helped us, for all the achievements Steve and I experienced while there—including the birth of our first child—Georgia would never feel like home.

After our wedding, I grew accustomed to my long days with the Social Security Administration. Sure, I cloaked some serious spasticity at times. But I did everything I could to guarantee I would offer optimum effort during the hours spent on the job. Most days I covered well, even when I felt tired, or drained, or completely exhausted and filled with spasticity. But one day, I began to wonder if I was losing control—if my condition was getting worse for some unknown reason. *I don't think I'm getting a cold or flu, I don't have my period, and I got a good night's sleep last night.* As I packed up my belongings at the end of my workday, I wasn't sure what to think. I grabbed my car keys and started my walk down the isle of cubicles to say goodnight to everyone I passed.

As I stepped into the warmth of the Georgia sun, I took a deep breath, and suddenly had to grab onto the railing of the steps outside the Social Security Administration building. My balance was off and each step I took made me feel like I was carrying two of me. Halfway to my car I stumbled and fell to the black pavement. Shaking, I fumbled to my feet as quickly as I could. *I hope no one saw me.* I looked ahead and saw Fred, a co-worker, in his white car. He put his friendly face out the window and asked, "You okay?"

"Yeah, I'm fine," I replied with a smile, even though I was completely bothered by the fact that I fell in public.

Fred persisted, "You need help getting to your car?"

"No, I'm okay … just a little clumsy." I assured him that I was all right, and thanked him as I ventured to my own car. Finally within fob range, I hit the little button on my key chain to unlock my driver's side door. Although the keyless remote was not standard with a Mercury Sable back then, I was thankful for my parents' early college graduation gift, given to me three years prior to the move to Georgia.

Sensing the urgency to use the bathroom, I bolted through my front door. Within a few minutes, I fought to get my pants up so I could crawl onto my bed to wait for Steve. I closed my eyes. *What is going on with my body? Maybe I'm pregnant.* I reviewed all the possible reasons why my coordination and balance would be this bad. *I'm not sick, and I have been sleeping really well. I don't have my period … on second thought, I should have my period.*

We ate out for dinner that night, so I finally took a moment to tell Steve, "Something isn't normal with my body." I explained to him my balance issues. "I fell on the way to the parking lot today. I wonder if I'm pregnant." He reminded me that I always say this when I have a bad day and "it's never because you're pregnant." Shortly after we left the restaurant, Steve pulled into Kmart and parked his white Dodge Ram.

"What are you doing?" I asked him as he hopped out of the truck.

"Getting you a pregnancy test," he said as he shut the door.

After a few minutes in the truck alone, I watched Steve as he exited the store with a small plastic bag in hand. He threw it on the seat between us. "Here," he said, looking at his purchase. "This should put an end to you thinking you're pregnant," he chuckled.

Shortly after we got home, Steve asked if I had taken the test yet.

"No," I replied. "The instructions on the box state that you should take the test with your first urine flow of the day."

"Whatever," he said, and we didn't discuss it the rest of the night.

I woke at 5:30 A.M., looked at the clock, and concluded I was done sleeping. Knowing that there was a pregnancy test waiting for me in the bathroom, I suddenly felt the full force of my bladder. *How can I sleep? I gotta go.*

I got out of bed, found the Kmart bag, then opened the box for complete instructions. *Really? How hard can it be to pee on a stick? Plus sign means I'm pregnant. Minus sign, I'm not.* The instructions indicated that I must wait five minutes for the results. But before I had the chance to pull up my pants, a pink plus sign magically formed on the stick. *The plus sign must mean negative.* I fumbled with the box to look again at the instructions. Clearly printed in large lettering, the box spelled it out: "The Plus sign means you're pregnant!"

I must have looked at the stick wrong.

My head turned several times: I looked at the stick, then back at the box, then back to the stick again. *Wow … is it true this time? Is Steve gonna believe me?*

It's too early to wake him. I'll wait until he's up for work. I climbed back into bed and tried to fall asleep. Flat on my back, I searched for the right words—the exact way to share the news. I stared at the ceiling, as if the perfect phrase would scroll down for me. I got nothing.

As soon as the clock read 6:30, I cuddled up to Steve, hoping that my restlessness would wake him. *I can't hold the news in any longer.* He rolled onto his back and looked at me.

"I'm pregnant," I told him, alert and poised for his response. I'm sure my eyes bugged out as if I had downed a pot of coffee. But it wasn't caffeine that had me charged up. It was the news I couldn't wait to share with the man who doubted me the night before.

"What?" he asked. The look on his face told me that he thought he was dreaming.

"I'm pregnant."

"Are you sure?" he said, starting to sit up.

"Yes. I took the test."

"Go get the box," he said in disbelief, moving into a full upright position.

I retrieved the box and the stick, then climbed back onto the bed next to Steve, who now sat up with some interest. I gripped the white stick and extended my hand right under his nose. His eyes, looking considerably more alert by now, studied the stick closely.

"Hand me the instructions."

I did as I was told, and then watched as his eyes rolled from the box to the stick several times, as if he were watching a miniature game of tennis—just as I had done an hour earlier.

Finally, the tennis game stopped. Our eyes met, and we both slowly smiled with the synchronized thought, "We're going to have a baby."

My first concern kicked in just moments after the micro tennis game ended. I was on a lot of medication. *I know that I can take baclofen while pregnant, because that's what Dr. Anderson told me years ago.*

"I just don't know about these other medications," I told Steve— my way of asking him to help me manage the onset of this enormous responsibility. Neurontin, Valium, metoprolol. "I'm growing a baby in my body. I can't take a chance on having this child be abnormal just because I needed to take these medications." Steve agreed— I should stop taking everything but baclofen, at once.

I woke the next morning feeling ill. I ran to the bathroom and threw up anything that remained in my stomach from the day before. I walked to the kitchen to have a bowl of cereal, only to vomit it up moments after eating. *This is going to be a long nine months.*

In bed that night, I couldn't lie still. My limbs involuntarily spasmed, even when I put all my focus into staying calm. Then, every time Steve moved or rolled over in his sleep, my whole body became spastic. I held back my tears. *I can do this. I will do this. If I can put myself in this situation, I can get through it. I don't have a choice. I'm growing an infant in me. A helpless baby is depending on me to do the right thing. I'll eat right. I'll quit those medications. I will give up my daily Coke fix. I'll give this baby a great life.* The pep talks were incessant and filled hours of sleepless time in bed.

I never slept at all that first night after my pregnancy test. It wasn't because I was excited. It wasn't because of fear. It was because I felt like absolute crap. *This is ten times worse than any stomach virus I've ever had or could imagine having. I feel like if I died right here and now, it would be okay.*

I couldn't stop shaking in my bed, and the vomiting wouldn't stop either. The more I shook, the more I felt the urge to heave. I was punishing myself—I'm not sure why. Without a doctor's order, I stopped my medications cold turkey ... without knowing what I was in for ... without inquiring if this was truly in my baby's best interest. All kinds of crazy things went through my mind in that first twenty-four hours after seeing the pregnancy plus sign. In retrospect, I should have consulted a physician before taking things into my own hands. I might have prevented some unwarranted withdrawal, and dodged the worst self-scolding I have ever endured.

This is hell. I'm in a living hell ... I have to make this baby strong and healthy. This child isn't going to have deformities because I couldn't give up my meds. It was stupid chance that made me this way ... it wasn't anybody's fault that I'm spastic and disabled. But I'm not taking one risk that the same thing happens again ... I'll do everything I can to make life for my baby different. I can't control what God has planned, but I can control what I put in my body. From now on, there will be no more alcohol, no medication (other than baclofen), no caffeine ... no matter how much I think I want or need them.

I called in sick every day that week. I wavered back and forth between believing this baby was making me ill and the likelihood that drug withdrawal had attacked my body. Each day I woke up, vomited at least once ... often two or three times ... then battled with the idea of going to work. *I'm too weak to take a shower. I'm lucky if I got two hours of sleep again last night.*

This struggle went on all week. I couldn't sleep in the bed with Steve anymore, because every time he moved, I went into full-body spasm. I asked him to put one of the twin mattresses from the guest bedroom on our bedroom floor. I fidgeted and spasmed as much as I needed to, without disrupting Steve's night of sleep.

Then, on Thursday night, Steve called my boss, Randy Thompson, to inform him that I was still sick. *I know that everyone at work is probably gossiping about me. I feel so lousy, I really don't care what they*

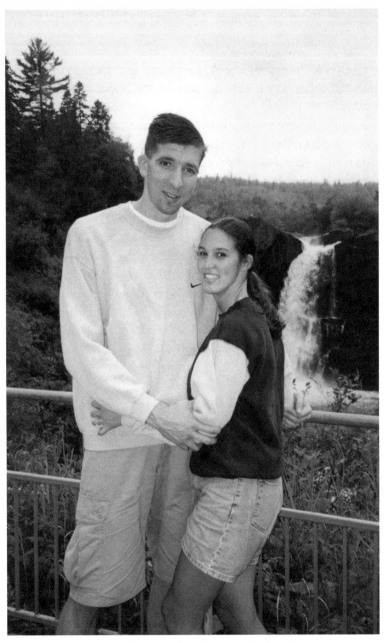

Jean and Steve on their honeymoon in Canada

have to say about me. I was definitely not myself. Whether it was withdrawal or the stress of carrying a baby, paranoia was winning. It was time for a doctor's attention.

By Friday morning, Steve was driving me to the office of an obstetrician. Exhausted, I had no control left. Steve had to do everything for me. At the clinic, he put me in a wheelchair since, with *or* without his help, I could no longer walk. The lack of sleep and medication withdrawal had taken its toll on me.

I felt my paranoia heighten as soon as I walked into the doctor's office, especially upon noticing a co-worker's wife waiting for her own appointment. *Great ... when I return to work next week, everyone in the office is going to know that I'm pregnant.* The stress of knowing this agitated me even more.

I heard my name called, and I was relieved to be wheeled away from the waiting room. Dr. Schneider was all smiles as he greeted me. This older gentleman with white hair and a thick white mustache was so gentle and kind with me.

"Actually, Jean, you really shouldn't be on baclofen while you're pregnant." Instead, he believed metoprolol would work for my tremors. "We put many of our patients on that for high blood pressure during pregnancy without side effects for the baby."

In addition, Dr. Schneider prescribed something new which would be safe throughout my pregnancy. Then he told me, "Come back in a month." Of course, the best directive he gave me that day was to relax. He definitely lessened my biggest worries, which worked like a drug. What a sweet man ... I'm lucky he was the first name I saw in the yellow pages.

Despite the medical attention, there still wasn't a day that I didn't throw up my breakfast. I knew that many women endured this to bring life into the world. *If that's all I have to deal with, I think I'll survive.* But work was very exhausting—worse than ever. Every morning I wondered, *Can I survive this even one more day?*

I did my best to multitask. I answered the phones and did paperwork at the same time. Yet, I felt my co-workers questioning my ability to do a good job. *I hate this ... they think I'm not pulling my weight.*

It was true that I had altered my duties somewhat. For instance, I wasn't able to work the front window anymore. Juggling the stressful situations that came unannounced at the window, plus running to make copies, and answer people's questions ... I no longer had the stamina to do such things. It was much easier on my body to handle the phones, and help the public in a different way.

One afternoon, I hung up the phone after a long call with a claimant, and looked up to see Carmen. I smiled at her and said hello.

"Hi, Jean. How are you doing?"

I'm not far into my pregnancy at this point. I answer honestly. "It's not easy, but I'm doing fine," I say with a sincere smile.

"Good," she said. Then, leaning forward she added, "You know ... you don't have to go through this. You have options." I was instantly offended ... here was one mother telling an expectant mother that it was okay to terminate a pregnancy.

"I want this baby," I said with fiery eyes. I felt tears welling up, but I refused to let her bully me into thinking I wasn't capable of being a working mom. *I have to do everything in my power to show her and every person working here that I can get through my pregnancy, and also be the best mother there is. This baby is a gift from God. A funny walk and a little morning sickness won't stop me.*

"Okay," she stated, with an attitude that seemed to say, "Well, I tried, but I can't get through to this silly woman."

Once Carmen walked away from my desk, a strong sadness hit my heart. *It's one thing for people to think that I'm making a mistake with my own life ... but to come to me and tell me that my baby shouldn't even be born—that's just the cruelest thing I could have heard.* I felt so horrible that day. I really didn't know what to do. And it wasn't long before this sadness turned into anger—much quicker than I thought possible.

By the end of each workday, I was so completely worn out that I could no longer walk on my own. In fact, as each shift ended, my co-worker Mary helped me finish for the day. She came to my desk, led me by the arm, and walked me to sign out. My hands refused to work by this time of the day, so Mary signed my shift card for me, then walked me to my car. As soon as I settled into my seat, she would shut the car door. She always gave me a big smile, and left me to drive myself home. I hated it.

I hated getting any help at all—I was so used to my independent ways back in Minnesota. But Mary meant well, and by this point in my pregnancy, I really didn't have a choice. Once I saw that Mary was focused on getting into her own car, I would begin my struggle to buckle up. It drove me insane that it took four to five tries to create enough force to pull the belt and buckle over my belly. Then I'd have to stop shaking long enough to find that stupid buckle slot. Sometimes I screamed in frustration as I gave the final pull. Like one of those tennis pros who grunt with each hit, the primordial scream seemed to do it. The metal would finally find the slot. *Click!* Exhaustion dictated my route home ... I would make no detours along the way. And although I was spent by the time I struggled through our front door, I still felt I had enough self-control to endure each day. I feared the time was coming when all self-control would be lost ... and a tiny, dependent infant would need me.

Finally, More Nice than Spice

A FEW MONTHS ALONG AND I WAS STILL NOT SHOWING, EVEN though my cravings heavily influenced my appetite. I still had trouble keeping down a bowl of cereal every morning. However, my ability to consume calories improved as each day progressed. Steve and I sat outside one evening and I watched him get the grill ready for burgers. He was drinking a beer and I had my glass of ice water.

"I'm getting hungry. I'll just have a little something to hold me over," I said as I stepped into the kitchen for a snack. I grabbed a can of green beans, opened it, dumped the entire can into a bowl, then stared at the front of the microwave as they heated up to a reasonable temperature. I heard the beep, grabbed the bowl, and joined Steve outside by the grill, popping beans into my mouth as if I had a bowl of popcorn. Steve tilted his head to the side and remarked, "I thought you'd come out with some chips to share." We both laughed, while I finished the whole can of beans—without sharing.

Almost every day after work, I went straight from the bathroom to the fridge. I craved a crisp, Claussen pickle—garlic, deli-style. When I bit into one, I finally understood what was meant by "comfort food." Suddenly, my drive home became easier because I knew that crispy crunch and salt were waiting for me. Then, rather accidentally, I discovered the perfect beverage pairing for my pickle. To wash down my salty treat nothing else would do but a big glass of apple juice.

"This is the best!" I said while Steve watched me savor every bite.

He looked up from the kitchen table—full of his MBA coursework—and gave me that look, like I had grown an extra head. Steve was immersed in his studies. He had quit his job in order to work full time on his master's in business administration. Our new plan: We would put the new house up for sale and move back to Minnesota once the baby was born. Despite our tight budget, Steve still gave me the green light to buy name-brand pickles! A sign of true love! Of course, I was the sole breadwinner now, and should have some say in the grocery list.

I knew we weren't going to be in Georgia for long, since Steve missed many things about the Midwest too. However, I never thought that he would formulate a plan to move to Minnesota. This was the one state in which he had earlier claimed he would never live.

"Iowa is fine," I remember him stating. But Minnesota just didn't thrill him. Somehow my home state's image changed, however, inviting him with opportunities to make a good living, and enjoy the outdoors—two important priorities for a man I knew would always be a good provider. Plus, it was only a five-hour drive from his family, and we both agreed our child should have the opportunity to know his or her grandparents, aunts, uncles, and cousins. Yet, the move would have to wait since Steve's master's coursework had to be completed in Georgia. This was a few years before online options, so with a lot already invested, Steve had to see the program through.

Soon apple juice wasn't enough. I needed every apple product on the market—McIntosh, Gala ... whatever variety of fresh apple I could find. And applesauce too. I was surprised that I craved healthy foods. I always heard that pregnant women demanded ice cream and chips. My vice was the Claussen pickle, but other than that, I was greedy for green beans and anything apple. Conversely, I hated chocolate. Every time I ate it, I could watch the clock and, within thirty minutes, expect to have a major call to the bathroom. My old favorite treat became poison. *I don't know if I can raise a child that doesn't like chocolate. I hope I get over this aversion.*

* * *

One day after work, while Laura walked me out, I unexpectedly tripped and landed on my right knee. *I have to get up before anyone else sees me.* I could tell I wasn't getting up quickly enough. I felt several eyes of the office staff on my back. Laura helped me to my feet, walked me to my car, and I assured her that I was fine. I smiled as she closed the door, even though I hated that the office staff buzzed behind my back. *They don't think I can handle this job. They don't think I should have a baby.* I had overheard a few co-workers talking: "Her stomach is really small. She's gonna end up with a one-pound baby." As hard as I tried to ignore people's doubts, my fall in the parking lot brought every gossipy thought to the forefront.

The gossip was real—not paranoia from my own doubts. Oliver reinforced this when he told me one day that he had "only weighed sixteen ounces when he was born."

"Really," I replied, wavering between anger that he felt I needed this information and gratitude that he cared enough to reassure me. *Essentially he's saying, small doesn't have to mean disaster … but your baby's clearly not growing right.*

I understood that Oliver was trying to help—to assure me that even if my baby was tiny, it could grow and be healthy too. What I really wanted, however, was for everyone to stop speculating … to be supportive. *Stop talking behind my back. You all talk about going to church every Sunday, having such Christian concern for the world. Well, prove it! Why not act a little more Christian and stop judging me. Is this how God wants us to behave? Is this what Jesus would do?* Of course, I didn't have the courage to say this out loud.

For these reasons and more, work was getting harder, but I focused on doing my job of answering the phones. Alma, the assistant manager, came to my desk one day and said that she needed to talk to me in Margaret's office. I walked with Alma into the district manager's office and Margaret gestured for me to sit across from her desk. I slowly got to the chair and collapsed into the seat.

Alma gave me a smile out of the corner of her mouth, then asked, "Did you hurt yourself or the baby yesterday when you fell?"

Immediately, my stomach churned, but looking at Alma, I felt as if she genuinely cared. I started shaking and felt the need to vomit. My face fell, but only for a moment. I found the motivation to perk up with a smile, and inform her, "I'm fine. No worries. You know … I can be kind of a klutz."

Margaret then proceeded to inform me (as an employee, not a concerned friend) that "we can't have anyone help you out to your car any longer. We'll arrange for a wheelchair and someone can push you out to the car for the time being." She suggested that Steve start driving me to and from work. She talked about my safety, but the translation in my head said, "You really shouldn't be here, and you certainly shouldn't be pregnant."

When Margaret suddenly switched to the topic of Steve … that *he* should be working rather than going to school … that *he* should be aware that a high-risk pregnancy is a big responsibility … I began to listen with precision again. "Pregnant, with a disability … this is a difficult thing."

An older woman—probably in her early sixties at that time— Margaret's own struggles to get ahead as a working woman within the Social Security Administration should have brought her to my defense. I was baffled by her scolding. She truly believed that I shouldn't have been working so hard.

I found the courage to say, "I don't mind working … I enjoy my job." But my defense was not very strong when put on the spot like that. I thanked them for their concern and walked back to my desk.

I plopped down in my chair and logged on to my computer. As I stared at my screen, tears began to sting in my eyes. *I will not cry. I will not cry. At least not here in the office.*

Mary must have seen me and sensed my stress, because she walked over to my desk.

"Are you okay?" she whispered as she rubbed my back with her hand.

I shook my head and replied, "No." Two tears dropped to my cheek. I explained what just happened in Alma's office and she looked at me with disbelief. She told me that she would be available to help me no matter what. "God will help you get through this time in your life, Jean. You're such a strong person." Mary knew exactly what to say that day. She gave me strength to get through that afternoon, and soon my hurt was turning into anger.

Many thoughts cluttered my mind for the rest of that shift. *I know that I'm doing my job. The phones are being answered and the public is being served by me in a timely manner. Margaret has no right to tell me that my husband should quit school and I should go home and wait for this baby to be born.*

With anger fueling my confidence, I decide to defend myself further. *I accept that no one in the office should have to walk me out to my car every day. But I'm not about to use a wheelchair, either.*

That night, Steve and I discussed the issue and decided that I should keep my scooter at work and get to my car using that. For the next two months, Brenda, another saving grace at my job, helped me get out to my car. At the end of each workday, she drove my scooter to my desk. I got on the scooter and then she led me outside, opening the doors so I could escape each night. She held the car door open for me and then closed it once I was inside. As soon as I was in the car, she jumped on the scooter, gave me a bright smile, and drove the thing back to my desk so it was ready for the next day. She didn't judge me. She didn't make me feel as if I was a burden to her. She just helped a friend get ready to do a good job for the day. Brenda proved something that every employee of the Social Security Administration should already have known—with a little bit of assistance, even a few obstacles will not stop a person's drive to be independent and work. Brenda was my blessing from God that helped me prove this. I counted on her help until the baby was born, and she never let me down.

In my final trimester, I began to fear that I shouldn't drive anymore, especially at the end of the workday. I was pretty exhausted, and my arms physically would not cooperate. "I just don't think it's safe for me to drive anymore," I told Steve. He agreed to start driving me to and from work every day. This took a load off my mind. *I know it is the right decision. I can't wait for this baby to be born. It is taking all of my energy, and making me feel dependent on others.*

At about seven months along, I was still not showing very much. My co-workers shared more and more concern that there was something wrong with my baby ... *why? Because I haven't gained fifty pounds and I don't have a huge basketball under my shirt?* To make matters worse, Susan—another co-worker who did indeed gain major weight, and did carry the big baby bump—gave birth to a five-pound newborn!

I called my mom after Susan's news, and she told me not to worry about it. "I was the same way. People didn't even know I was pregnant," she laughed. "And I had eight-pound babies." To hear her say this over the phone was very reassuring. After all these years, Mom's wisdom still calmed me. What a gift she had for saying just the right thing.

With the birth of this baby nearing, I spent more time with Dr. Schneider. Each and every checkup required a urine sample ... something with which Steve had to help me. Entering the bathroom together, I stood in front of the toilet and held onto the handicap arm rail as Steve pulled my pants down. After a long day of work, I just couldn't do it. *This is humiliating, but I don't have a choice.* I was able to hold the cup on my own, but when I finished, he had to pull my pants back up. *Not exactly the romantic encounter a husband expects when his wife returns from being at work all day.* In fact, my routine after work now was to crawl onto my bed ... not for some snuggling with my hubby, but for a ten-minute power nap before attempting to pee. Funny what long work hours and a final gestational period will do to a woman's libido.

One day I had to drive myself home from work for some reason. I knew I had to use the bathroom at the end of my workday, but decided to wait until I got to my own house. I went straight to the toilet this time, skipping my ten-minute nap. I had to go so badly, I started pulling at my black dress pants, but my useless fingers kept slipping down the fabric. I took a breath. *This just isn't going to happen.* I pulled and pulled, but my hands, shaking and devoid of all motor skills, felt as if I were wearing giant oven mittens. I had no grip, my pants weren't budging, and my lower torso burned in pain as my bladder was about to explode. *What the heck … I* surrendered to the pain. I sat down on the toilet, leaned forward, and peed with my pants on. Relief … and humiliation all at once. *Life isn't fair.*

I hate being pregnant and will be so happy when this is over. I'm finally showing. But this just makes getting around even harder.

"Well, the baby seems to be growing at a good pace," Dr. Schneider sounded positive. I think he knew he had to lead with some cheerleading since this was the day we discussed my labor.

"He seems to think I should have a C-section to make the birth easier," I told my mom on the phone that night. "But his associate thinks I would be better off having a vaginal birth." Actually, the two doctors had compromised. They agreed it would be best to induce me two weeks early. Before they would induce me, however, they would order an epidural. "As soon as they know the epidural is working, they're gonna induce me." This was a relief to me. I didn't mind being deprived true labor pains. Plus, I didn't want a C-section. *This plan is good.*

I have about one month to go and then this baby will be out of me and I will be a mother. Dr. Schneider was so supportive, but finally voiced concern about one thing. It was just brought to his attention that metoprolol could cause low birth weights. I looked over at Steve, begging for reassurance. *I have done so much to deliver a healthy baby.* I bowed my head and said to myself, *Please, Lord, this baby has to be healthy.*

"I'd like to get a look at a sonogram, Jean," Dr. Schneider explained. "Just a precaution … just so we can plan if necessary." The room down the hall was plain and empty with the exception of all of the medical devices. I lay back on the table and recalled all the babies in my hospital room back when I had my muscle transfer at age twelve. *I don't want my baby spending its first months in a hospital ward. Please, God, let me be like my mother, hiding a full-sized infant in this lean body of mine.*

The technician pulled my shirt up past my small belly and squirted a cool, clear jelly on my baby bump. She took the sonogram camera and placed it on the cool jelly and spread it around while I looked at the monitor to my right. *I see my beautiful baby. It's in there.* I looked at Steve, and smiled with relief. Then the technician showed us where the heart was, and all the fingers, toes, and a pretty big head. I noticed Steve smiling as we studied the monitor.

"The baby's weight looks good. Looks over six pounds for sure," she said smiling at each of us. Many thoughts of gratitude went through my head. *Thank you, God. Thank you!* I continued to look at my amazing baby on the screen, and I spotted its hand up by its mouth.

"The baby's sucking its thumb," the technician said, pointing at the precise spot on the monitor. "I'll print a picture of that for you," she said, pressing buttons on her computer. She continued to move the camera around my stomach and stopped to ask, "Do you want to know the sex?"

"No," I said.

"Yes," Steve answered simultaneously.

We looked directly at one another. "I don't want to know if it's a boy or a girl. I want to be surprised," I explained.

"This happens a lot," the technician stated. "I can write it on a piece of paper." She reached for a notepad. "Steve can look at it and you can still be surprised." I wasn't thrilled with this offer.

"That will never work. I can't have him knowing the sex of the baby when I don't know. He'll slip and tell me what it is."

Steve defended himself. "I won't slip. I can keep it a secret."

"No way. If you're going to know, then I want to know too." I took a deep breath and flustered, I announced, "Fine, tell us what we're having."

The technician needed confirmation that we both wanted to know. "Yes," I agreed, but also informed Steve, "This will not happen with our next baby."

"You're going to have a girl," she smiled and patted my shoulder.

I looked at her and then Steve in disbelief. *We're going to have a girl. A healthy girl that will be at least six pounds.* I was ecstatic, even though I didn't get my way. The technician cleaned up my stomach, lowered my shirt and helped me sit up. I got off the table and walked out of the clinic holding onto Steve. I was not just a pregnant woman, but the mom of a daughter.

"Sugar and spice, and everything nice" ... the old saying went off in my head. *I have felt everything but nice toward my doubting co-workers.* I decided to share my news at the office instead of having them speculate behind my back.

"I'm having a girl!" I could see that they were genuinely happy for me. I learned that they planned a baby shower for me the following week. "Yeah—girl gifts! What fun!" someone announced.

I knew that no one wished harm for me or the baby, but those months as a pregnant employee brought such a strain to me as I became the object of office drama. I wondered if people realized how easy it was to detect their disapproval. Well, at least that day when I announced the gender, I felt sincere support for a healthy baby girl.

Within days, my body felt different. My muscles weren't contracting like they had been for the past eight months. Walking became easier again. In fact, I was able to walk to the bathroom and to lunch without help. Dr. Schneider said, "That's normal. A pregnant woman's body often relaxes at the end of a pregnancy." I wasn't going to argue with such good news ... plus, it seemed to indicate that I could go anytime.

As I walked toward the exit at the end of the day, Carmen stopped me in the hall. "I just want you to know that you are the most beautiful pregnant woman that I have ever seen. I'm sorry for what I said before," she added as she gave me a hug.

"Thanks," I said, hugging her in return. It didn't erase the pain from our earlier conversation. But it helped me to know that she regretted her negative words. *It had to be difficult for her to say this. She would not have said anything if she didn't really mean it.* Just as Dr. Schneider suggested, all the stress my body had been feeling seemed to be fading ... and along with it, my mistrust of others who had questioned my decision to carry a baby. The knowledge that I would soon be holding a precious baby girl made my last month of pregnancy my easiest.

Winona, Old Faithful, and Other Maternal Matters

THE BIG DAY HAD ARRIVED! WE WERE INSTRUCTED TO MEET Dr. Schneider at the Coliseum Medical Center by 10:00 A.M. I was feeling very hungry, but couldn't eat until after the baby was born. C-section potential was still real. I didn't want to even think about it, but agreed to the typical precautions anyway. The epidural frightened me enough. One visual I tried to block from my morning thoughts—a needle in my spine—still beat the alternative of emergency surgery. *Come on, Baby Girl—cooperate, would ya?!*

As Steve and I walked into the hospital, I had one thought on my mind: *If all goes well, we will be parents in a few hours.*

"Change into this gown. I'll be back in a few minutes." The nurse gave me directions to climb into the hospital bed. Once I had changed out of my clothes, my vitals were taken and all of my medical information was typed into the computer. Thirty minutes later, the anesthesiologist arrived to give me the epidural.

My nerves were a dead giveaway—I dreaded this step.

"You have to relax," the doctor said as he sat on the bed beside me. "Here, let's have you sit on the edge ... and Steve, stand in front of Jean. Hold her hands. Yep, like that."

The doctor rubbed some warming alcohol on my back and told me to take a few deep breaths. After a slight pinch of pain ... we were done. Steve and the doctor helped me swing my legs back into the bed. *Now, we just have to wait for everything to go numb. Then Dr. Schneider can get things started.*

Once induced, I immediately noticed a change—a complete lack of activity. If it hadn't been for the monitor, I don't think I would have felt at all involved in the event that made everyone else so attentive. Laura, my mentor from work, called just as an enormous contraction took place on the screen. "How are you doing?"

With a smile on my face I replied, "Great! I've had three contractions since you've called!" Steve still teases me that while Winona worked to come into the world, I spent the day watching Oprah.

The nurses checked my cervix throughout the late afternoon. I still hadn't eaten, but the IV in my arm took care of my hunger pains.

"Things are coming along nicely." I grew confident with each positive report. *This has to be the easiest day of my pregnancy. I can't believe I worked through yesterday.* I doubt if many of my co-workers believed I would work until the day my labor kicked in.

Later that evening, the nurse reported that I had dilated to seven. "It will be a few more hours. We're looking at a little after midnight, so rest if you can." I closed my eyes. *If she's born tomorrow, her birthday will be 2/2/2002. It will be easy to remember that!*

The checks became more frequent—it was hard to sit back and relax. So when the nurse assessed me less than half an hour later and announced, "It's time," I shot into ready position. *This baby wants February 1 for her birthday!*

Dr. Schneider appeared from the air, or so it seemed. My boring hospital room now had the energy of my favorite ER episode. I had a nurse on my right arm and Steve on my left. Dr. Schneider guided my legs up to what felt like starter blocks for labor. Time to push. *They all want a sprint, not a marathon. I hope Coach gets his way.*

Dr. Schneider counted me down to my official first push. All we're missing is the sound of the pistol and him shouting, "On your mark! Get set! Go!" *Okay, I think I'm pushing, but I can't feel anything for sure.*

"Try again, Jean. Push!"

I was as compliant as could be—with all my strength, I gave it my best again. *This has to do it!*

"One more strong push!" Dr. Schneider commanded. I sensed that he wanted this over ASAP, and not necessarily for *my* sake.

Simultaneous with the next "push" order, he told the nurse to also push down on my stomach. Dr. Schneider had placed a suction cup on the baby's head. As I pushed, he pulled, and the nurse applied pressure to my abdomen. Dr. Schneider reprimanded the nurse for my tear which would require stitches, but the baby was out. They rushed her over to the corner of the room—checking her Apgar scores and cleaning her up.

I lifted my head off the table to see what they were doing with my baby—Steve and the nurses hovered over her. Moments later, the most beautiful baby I have ever seen was placed in my arms. I looked into her dark brown eyes—she was already looking intently back at me. *Welcome, Winona Jean Abbott.* All the drama of the pregnancy—all the worries of proving myself at work—all the struggles to be pregnant with a disability … suddenly forgotten. *This is the secret joy I was missing! This is God's greatest gift to me. Welcome to my world, Winona!*

* * *

"Does she have any hair?" My mom asked a logical question on the phone that night, but I somehow had forgotten to look under Winona's newborn cap to see. It would be some hours before I could answer with a confident "yes." *What kind of mother allows her baby to be whisked away without careful inspection?* This would be the first of many moments when I felt under-qualified as a parent. One nurse told me, "Get used to it."

Both of my parents were surprised by *granddaughter* Winona, but for very different reasons. Back before my Dad knew the gender of our baby, he went so far as to purchase and mail us a blue musical bear for his unborn baby *grandson*. When the gift arrived, I could hear Dad saying, "It's just gotta be a boy!" When we learned the gender from the ultrasound image, my mom refused to be told. Dad, on the other hand, let us share our new knowledge. He waited patiently for the moment of truth. Now, wrapped in a pink blanket, Winona was officially ours. *I don't think Dad will doubt his baby granddaughter is the perfect package he's been waiting for.*

Steve's brother, stationed in South Carolina, and his sister in Michigan, drove great distances to see and hold Winona. They didn't stay long—I'm sure Steve gave them the memo that I wanted space and time to heal, and to adjust to taking care of our baby's needs. I had focused on my own care for so long … concerns for healthy sleep, managing my baclofen, house chores that took extra time, etc. Now, I had the unknown factors of motherhood thrown into the mix. *Would Winona keep us up all night? Would she eat and grow like she should? Or would I have to wrestle with her health, too?* Mom eased many of my worries, and guided us into a routine, but the mix of anxiety and excitement in those first few weeks made me want to post a sign on our front door: *Unless you are Mom or Steve, stay away … until I get this figured out.* Fortunately, everyone seemed to understand and respect this.

Mom arrived in Macon the day we were discharged, and I had two solid weeks of attentive help from the best nurse ever. Dad's delayed drive to Georgia to retrieve his wife meant he would finally meet Winona. With the start of her third week in the world, my parents kissed Winona goodbye, pulled out of our driveway, and made the road trip back to Minnesota … a mini-vacation for them. I'm sure I cried the day they left. Going solo for the first time in my mommy role terrified me. My mother's parting words: "You'll do great!"

Steve's dad waited until graduation day to meet Winona. Once Steve finished his MBA, we could make our move back home, and Lynn would be indispensable. Winona loved meeting her other grandpa, and we couldn't have finalized the move without him.

* * *

Soon after Mom and Dad left, we stopped by my office to share our good news with everyone.

"She's adorable!"

"Look at that hair!"

"You look great! What did she weigh?"

"Seven pounds, nine ounces—and nineteen-and-a-half inches long."

"Wow! Good-sized baby!"

"I know—we're so lucky. Thanks."

This visit was so fun! The stress of being a working parent would not hit me for a while.

Motherhood quickly became the greatest paradox of my life. *How could something be so challenging and so rewarding at the same time? I don't see myself getting bored in the next eighteen years. In fact, I would highly welcome boredom.*

At six weeks old, Winona watched me go back to work. I wanted to stay home with her forever, but it was official. Our house went up for sale and our plot to move back to Minnesota was contingent upon Steve's MBA from Mercer University. Leaving Winona each morning to go to work was torture, but knowing the end was near—

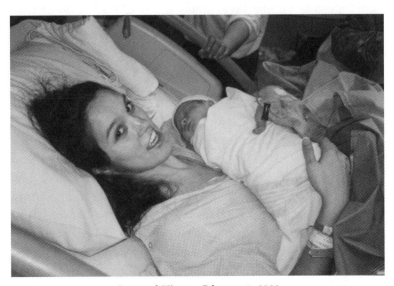

Jean and Winona, February 1, 2002

that close family and friends would soon be back in our lives—made things tolerable. Our hope was that Winona's cousins would be like siblings to her, and that every happy holiday and event would be spent with them. I was eager to spend time with these kids as well. It was hard to believe that Mike and Tom each had two children—I felt so far removed from them. I looked forward to our move home to Minnesota for so many reasons.

My days at the Social Security office were tiring, but I enjoyed my job and always felt as though I made a difference in other people's lives. However, when four o'clock hit, I had no interest in overtime anymore. I made my way to my car as fast as I could, so I could spend the rest of the day with Winona.

Most days, I opened the door of our home to have Steve hand off the baby so he could gather his things for campus. Five nights a week he had class either at the Macon or the Atlanta campus. He left us just before dinner and rolled back home sometime after 11:00 P.M.

It never failed that when Steve opened the door to the garage to leave for his commute, my heart fell, and a sad, sick feeling crept in. I knew deep down that I was quite capable of staying home with Winona—feeling like a single mother in the evenings was only temporary. And I often thought about couples who did this regularly, who perhaps worked different shifts to avoid having the expense of daycare—couples who gave up their time together for the greater financial good of the family. When I heard the mechanical sound of the garage door closing, I knew that it was just Winona and me for yet another night. This lonely, blue feeling would only last a few more weeks. I couldn't wait for Steve's graduation!

"How's my girl?" I asked, carrying Winona over to the love seat. I sat and played with her, ignoring the thought that I had no one to call—no one to share her with all evening. It was not like me to live without close friends, but my time in Georgia had not been conducive to making connections like I had back home. Baby Winona distracted me from analyzing this change in my life. Clearly, she was worth it! I couldn't take my eyes off of her.

So beautiful... when she smiled, she looked so much like Steve.

"You look like Daddy! Yes, you do!" I wondered if she thought, *But Daddy says I look like you!*

Steve was convinced that she looked so much like me. I guess he couldn't get past her coloring. Winona had my olive skin, my dark hair, and my big brown eyes that today are even a little bit darker than mine. However, her features were so much like Steve's ... the shape of her eyes and the curve of her mouth ... I loved that she was a true combination of the two of us.

For at least a half hour every night, I sang songs to Winona. I remembered my mom sitting with me on the living room couch, singing songs like, "Baa, Baa, Black Sheep" and "Twinkle, Twinkle, Little Star." I loved hearing my mom's voice and having her undivided attention. I wanted Winona to look back and remember me singing to her too.

I was usually exhausted by the time I finished my own dinner, so I hopped into my pajamas and turned on the television, mostly for some noise. I held Winona out, my arms extended. She loved when I put her face up to mine, smiled at her, then gently bobbed her up and down. Her smiles back at me warmed my heart.

As time passed, she would get fussy. Winona rarely cried, but since the clock read 6:55, I knew she was both hungry and tired. I left her on the floor so I could make her evening bottle in the kitchen. Most people would think it a little early for a nighttime bottle, but since I took longer to prepare everything, I had to time a feeding just right. I learned this the hard way. I knew what would happen if I let my baby get too hungry. I knew that I could not let my disability keep me from prepping a bottle like other moms could.

I grabbed an empty bottle from the cupboard above the sink. In order to do this, I actually had to hold onto the kitchen counter to keep my balance and prevent a fall on the linoleum. Next, I grabbed the large container of formula and ladled three scoops of cream-colored powder into the bottle. I screwed the cap and nipple onto the bottle, placed my finger over the hole and shook it for ten seconds to mix it all well. Slowly, I dragged my feet back into the living room, sat down on the couch, and leaned over my baby girl squawking on the floor.

"Are you hungry?" I asked as I propped the bottle against the couch so it didn't leak. "I'm sorry it takes mommy so long to get your bottle ready." I bent over to pick up Winona. Her curling lip made the cutest pout as she cried.

"Come here, fussy baby." I position her thick black hair in the crook of my left arm, which rested on the arm of the couch.

"Here we go, Winona," I said as I grabbed the bottle and placed it in her mouth. She went after it as if she hadn't had a thing to eat all day. She was a really good eater and I knew that she had probably had several six-ounce bottles while I was at work that day. She continued to drink quickly and her eyes began to grow tired. Her sucking seemed to slow down, but I saw that she had only taken half of her bottle.

I pulled the bottle from her mouth and carefully placed her head on my right shoulder. She was not easy to burp. I patted her back a few times and had poor results. I raised her up a little higher on my chest hoping that a touch more pressure would cause her to burp. A few more pats and a burp exploded. "Oh, my, baby girl! You sound like one of those Winona State college boys who just left the bar after too many beers!"

Actually, I was relieved. "All this belching and no spit up—success!" I said, kissing her head.

I positioned Winona on the floor and scooted myself down from the couch to sit next to her. *It's time for her diaper change.* I found that if I did this partway through her final bottle, she would wake up a little bit, and find the energy to finish her bottle. Diaper changes were one of my least favorite things to do as a mom. It wasn't because of the obvious. It was simply one of the most difficult things for me to physically do as a mother.

I didn't have any trouble undoing the snaps of her sleepers. It was everything else. Pay attention next time you change a baby. You actually need to use both hands simultaneously to change a diaper, and I could barely move one hand or arm, not to mention two in sync. The simple task of unfolding the diaper, then lifting her bottom off of the pad to slide the diaper under her was tricky. I feared I wouldn't get her little cheeks up high enough to slide the diaper into place. Folding the top of the diaper over her wasn't hard, but fastening the tabs on either side was. Getting things fastened on each side was a total frustration. The last thing I wanted was a leaky diaper, which could mean I would have to change her clothes too.

Not a day went by that I didn't thank God for the times I was living in. I couldn't imagine this job before disposable diapers. The laundry alone could have kept me working all night—but imagine me trying to secure safety pins! My hands were so shaky and unpredictable—I would have poked my fingers for sure. And Winona's bottom would have been like a pincushion!

With her diaper securely on, I attempted to button up the bottom portion of her sleeper. One by one, I fumbled with each and every snap. I couldn't believe that she cooperated while her mother took forever to get her ready for another night's sleep. I closed the last snap and sighed. *Okay—I am more than halfway done getting her ready for bed.*

I stayed seated on the floor, put Winona in my arm, grabbed the bottle that I had set just beside me, and inserted the nipple into her mouth again. She began to down the rest of the formula, and before long, she had finished all but the last couple drops in the bottle. I placed her on my shoulder and was surprised by her dainty burp. But a burp's a burp, so I lay her on the floor in front of me and grabbed a blanket for her. That's when it all went downhill.

She exploded like Old Faithful. The formula that I had worked so hard to make and deliver was all over the front of her sleeper. I took the burp cloth and desperately tried to wipe it off of her, but she was drenched. *The whole bottle must have come up.* It didn't seem to faze her, but I was a sad wreck. *I am going to have to change her again!* And it seemed impossible, but I felt I had to give her another bottle. I looked at her beautiful face and began to sob.

I was exhausted! Just when I thought I was almost done and close to getting myself to bed, I knew that I needed to start this whole ordeal over again. My tears kept falling. *I really don't know if I have it in me to do this again. Not tonight, anyway.* I took a long, deep breath and forced myself off of the floor and walked to the kitchen to make her another bottle, one hour after I started her original feeding.

My tears finally stopped and I struggled to get her out of the formula-soaked clothes. I gave her another bottle and changed her diaper, just in case. When all was done, I wrapped her in a blanket, and placed her on the floor, where she would sleep until Steve returned later that night. I always wondered, *Was I a bad mom for not putting my baby in her crib once she went to sleep?* Tonight was no different. I felt terrible that I couldn't lift my own child to place her in the crib and tuck her in for the night.

I called my mom. In those first few weeks after Winona was born, Mom had seen to it that I took a nap every day. She helped me with my sitz baths and advised me on what to do for hemorrhoids. She even helped me change my blood-stained maxi pads. These were not my finer moments in life, but she didn't seem to mind one bit.

All mothers know how sleep-deprived you can get when caring for an infant. It's not easy. My mom acknowledged this even more since she knew it had to be worse when faced with all the challenges of a neurological muscle disorder. She understood that physically I got much worse if I didn't get proper sleep. By the time Mom's two weeks with us were up, my little Winona was sleeping through the night. I'm not sure if I've ever heard of another baby doing that so soon after birth. I know that God doesn't give us more than we can handle, so I assume He must think that I really needed my sleep. I appreciated that.

Like a child, I needed my mother, more than I had in years. Every morning I woke, I thanked God that we were one day closer to moving back to Minnesota. *A day doesn't go by that I don't miss my mom.* She gave Winona her first bath and drilled it into my head that I should "feed the baby, then lay the baby down." Some may think you should hold a baby until she falls asleep, but the way Mom taught me actually trained Winona to fall asleep on her own. Good advice for every new mom! My mom was genius about this.

That night on the phone from Minnesota, she listened to my frustrations. I asked her if it was bad that I didn't carry my baby to her crib. As usual, Mom made me feel so much better.

"Jean. She is fed, she has clean clothes and a clean diaper, and most of all, she is safe and loved. She is perfectly fine where she is until Steve comes home." With that, I was able to turn off the living room light and put myself to bed.

"Goodnight, Winona. I love you." I flipped the switch and left my baby in the dark.

My Angel in the Sky

WINONA IS THREE MONTHS OLD TODAY AND THE TWO OF US ARE *flying home to Minnesota … for good!* As excited as I was to move back to the Midwest, I fretted over the flight. Steve would not be there to help with Winona. He and his dad needed to transport three vehicles—Steve's truck and my car hitched to the back of a loaded U-Haul—north from Macon.

My parents had intervened when they realized we faced a three-day road trip with all of our stuff. "Let us pay for your flight—you and Winona can fly home ahead of the guys."

With gratitude, I accepted the gift … despite the fear of three hours in the air with a baby on my lap. *If she cries the whole time, what will I do? It's not like I can take a walk with the stroller, or rock her to sleep after a few ounces of formula.* My typical tricks for Winona's crying jags—my favorite was to hand her off to Steve—would be impossible at an altitude of 30,000 feet. But this was our plan, and departure day had finally come.

Steve dropped Winona and me at the curb outside Hartsfield-Jackson International Airport. Before he drove away, he retrieved an airport wheelchair for me, then asked an employee to help me check my bag.

"Can you see that they are wheeled to the right area for takeoff?"

I had only one suitcase for essentials to survive the week without Steve. Formula, bottles, four sleepers and a couple of outfits for Winona … two pairs of jeans, a few tops, and a week's worth of underwear for me.

"There's not much space anyway—the less you bring, the better," my mom had warned me on the phone.

Moving is always a challenge, but we chose the absolute worst time to ask my folks if we could bunk with them while we searched for a home in Minnesota. My parents were in the middle of remodeling their house. The kitchen had been totally gutted of cupboards and appliances. There was no kitchen sink … no flooring.

"It's really torn up, but we'll make do."

How bad can it be? Who had endured more adversity than my parents, raising three busy kids, and dealing with my bed in the family room after my surgery? "It'll be fine, Mom. Hopefully, we'll find a new place fast."

Then Mom informed me that my brother and his family had moved in as well.

"Mike and Cathy sold their house quicker than they thought possible. They are staying here while they search too."

Mike and Cathy had the "bear room" … a guest bedroom with a crib for Jack, their ten-month-old. Sophia was sleeping in my old bedroom.

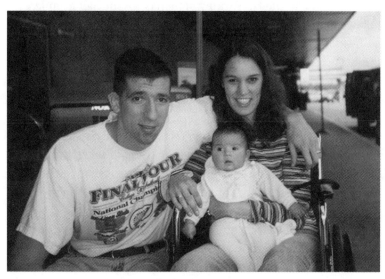

Steve, Jean, and Winona at the Atlanta airport

193

"You, Steve, and Winona will have to stay in the basement." This proved how eager I was to move my baby girl out of Georgia. Without hesitation I thanked my mom and said, "We'll make it work." I was optimistic that all was not as bad as the picture she had painted.

On the curbside, with Winona on my lap, Steve made one more request of the airport attendant: "Will you take a picture of us?"

This was the first time that we would spend multiple days apart, and Steve knew I hated to leave without him. He kneeled down next to my chair, put his arm around me, and we posed for our first family photo, just moments before I was pushed down the concourse. The picture was snapped, Steve kissed both his girls, and then he rushed off to finalize our permanent departure from Georgia.

Just as Steve opened the car door to leave, I looked down to see that Winona's pastel pink sleeper was wet from the bottom of her diaper up to the middle of her spine.

"Steve!" I all but jumped out of the wheelchair. "I need help changing her diaper. She's soaked through her clothes."

"I can't help," he said, holding the car door open. "I can't park here any longer."

He pointed to the No Parking sign, flashed me half a smile, and followed it up with, "I love you."

I watched as Steve climbed into the Buick and pulled away with the airport traffic.

Before I could do a thing for Winona, the airport employee began wheeling my chair. *How am I going to do this? I have to change Winona—diaper and clothes—before we take off.*

Winona sat back in my lap and relaxed for the ride. We made it through security, and were approaching the gate, when the woman wheeling us stopped to say, "When your plane is ready to board, a Delta employee will come for you." She put the brakes on my chair, just as I said, "Thank you."

Fearing the need for a quick change, I held Winona out in front of me so I could shimmy myself to the edge of my wheelchair. I grabbed the changing pad and laid it on the floor in front of me, thankful that the chair's brakes seemed secure. Placing Winona on the pad, I tried not to think of the germs hiding in the carpet fibers from daily traffic that crossed an airport floor. I slid out of the chair and down to the ground with Winona. From my bag, I dug out a clean yellow sleeper, a fresh diaper, and her wipes.

Here it comes. The stress from the situation triggered spasticity in my muscles. I blocked out the gawkers who sat around me. I felt their stares as my shaking hands began unsnapping Winona's wet sleeper. *Lord, please give me the strength and courage to get through this day. If I focus on getting Winona cleaned up, I won't shake as much.*

I noticed the clock on a nearby wall. *We have about an hour and a half before our flight takes off.* This information eased my nerves. *It could be worse—I could be doing this on the plane. This will be her last diaper change before we land in Minneapolis.* My pep talk was working—my shaking was fading.

Great! Of all the times . . . Winona was not only wet, she had pooped up her back. As ridiculous as it sounds, I stuffed my urge to say to my child, "Of all times to do this! What were you thinking, Winona? Really? At the airport?" Fortunately, I came to my senses before these words escaped my mouth. With a trembling fist full of wipes, I cleaned her up as best I could without dousing her in a bathtub.

Winona was so busy looking at her new surroundings she made this one of the easiest diaper changes ever! I noticed the clock again. *Record time—less than five minutes.* For some, that would seem like an eternity. For me, it was a blessing in a bad situation. I was learning to keep my cool. *I hope I have the same luck keeping you happy on the flight home.*

Winona and I stayed on the floor. *Why sit in a chair for any longer than we have to . . . two and a half hours in a tight airplane seat will be challenge enough.* Two women—I'd say in their mid-thirties, probably moms themselves—walked toward us.

Leaning over, they smiled at Winona and said, "If you need any help, just let us know."

I wish I could take them up on this. I could really stand to use the bathroom before I get on that plane. Using the bathroom alone can be challenge enough for me . . . I knew I could never accomplish it with

Winona in my arms. But I wasn't about to hand my baby off to complete strangers—I didn't care how trustworthy and sincere they seemed.

"Thanks, we're doing fine," I replied with a smile. *All those times I've had to hold my urine … at school … at work … on a bus or car ride … today will be no different. Add plane ride to the list.*

An hour into our wait, I heard a female voice announce over the loud speaker, "Minneapolis is running an hour behind." I looked down at the floor. *Winona, will this ever end? I definitely won't be drinking any soda or juice on this flight.*

Some time went by, and I shimmied up into my wheelchair again, Winona in my arms. I looked at the clock. Thankfully, it was nearly time to board. Winona sat alert and content. People-watching was definitely one of her favorite pastimes. *How is she going to handle it when I am the only face she sees for almost three hours?*

I recalled past flights where babies cried the entire time up in the air. I was prepared to give her a bottle during takeoff and landing to prevent her little ears from popping. However, I wasn't sure how she would handle sitting on my lap for the two hours in between. *Please, let there be a woman sitting next to me.*

My past experiences sandwiched between men on planes had been less than friendly. They generally wanted nothing to do with the person next to them, especially a child. No small talk—no armrest sharing. Once, Tom and I had seats by a big guy wearing a suit and tie. Yikes—a businessman seated with two kids who couldn't wait to get to Disney World in Orlando! He rolled his eyes as he sat down, implying he had been positioned next to the brattiest kids onboard. Subconscious or deliberate, I'm not sure—but Tom and I fulfilled his prophesy by playing cards and laughing all the way to Florida. At one point, Tom accidentally knocked his Coke off the tiny food tray and it landed right on the man's suit pants. Tom looked from me to the businessman and began to apologize profusely. The man soaked up the spill with a napkin, never looking at us or saying a word.

I cannot have a man sit next to me on this flight. I have been given enough challenges on this airport adventure. It would be really nice to sit next to a caring woman who understands exactly how long this day has been for me.

"Boarding has begun," the Delta employee alerted everyone waiting for the Minneapolis flight.

Panic struck. *They were supposed to put me and Winona on that plane before anyone else. How could they forget?* More importantly, how was I going to get past everyone else now crowding the line to find their seats?

I looked around to see if a Delta person was walking my way. *Nope—every employee is caught up in helping the line-up of passengers.*

We have to get on that plane, Winona. "We have to get on that plane!"

"Excuse me," I said, leaning out of my chair. The young woman trying to join the line thankfully looked my way. "Can you please ask one of the Delta employees to help me board the plane?"

She nodded her head and told me she'd be happy to get help for me. *I really hope I sit next to her. She seems kind and patient. Maybe she likes babies.*

A Delta employee came my way and apologized for making us wait.

"We will get you on this plane right now," she said. She released the brake on my chair and wheeled us to Winona's first flight.

"Can you walk to your seat once we enter the aisle, or will you need to be carried?"

I informed her that I could get myself to my seat—*I hate having to ask this*—"but I'll need you to carry my baby for me."

I found my aisle seat in a row of three and buckled myself in. The flight attendant handed me Winona. Then she placed my black diaper bag under the seat directly in front of me.

"Thank you so much," I said, trying to cover the anxiety I felt over the two empty seats left in my row.

A woman who appeared to be traveling by herself stopped at my aisle. I smiled at her. *I really hope you are sitting next to me.* She greeted me, stepped around me, and took the seat next to the window.

One seat down, one to go. Please, let it be a woman.

I sensed someone in the aisle, waiting for the middle seat. I looked up to see a man in his mid-thirties storing his carry-on just above me. He stepped carefully around Winona and me, sat, then buckled in.

You have got to be kidding. I leaned back in my seat, trying to relax as best I could. I took a deep breath, but I knew that Winona sensed my uneasiness. She began to fuss. I got her bottle ready for takeoff. I was sure that this would be the longest flight of our lives … especially for the man sitting next to me.

Takeoff went better than expected. Winona drank her bottle … *I don't think your ears even popped.* I could tell, however, she was tired of Mommy's face. Who could blame her … we had been at this for hours already, and the flight had just begun.

"She's beautiful. How old is she?" I was startled as the gentleman next to me seemed to strike up a conversation. *Wow—he's talking to us. He's asking about my baby girl.* She was definitely fussing, but he didn't seem bothered by it at all.

"Well, this is Winona, and she is three months old today," I answered with a smile. "She should be full and ready for a nap. But she's not about to fall asleep if she thinks she might miss something important, like looking at you."

The man made more small talk … then he began to make silly faces at Winona. She loved it! Smiling and cooing, she was finally beginning to relax—and so was I. He even played peek-a-boo with her. *What a relief! This guy really likes little kids.*

Winona couldn't seem to take her eyes off the man. "Would you mind if I held her?" he said, turning his attention to me.

Yikes—hand my baby over to a complete stranger?

While these cautious thoughts hid behind my smile, I also considered: *We are thirty thousand feet up in the air. This man isn't going anywhere.*

I handed Winona over to him, and he entertained her for the next hour and a half. *I know she likes to socialize, but this is insane.*

I could not get over how lucky I was to have this man sitting next to me.

A pilot interrupted Winona's amusement. "Please buckle up for landing" … my cue to make another bottle.

I informed Winona's new friend that I needed to give her a bottle "so her ears don't pop."

"Would you mind if I fed her?" he asked, informing me that both of his kids were teenagers. "My baby years are long gone. I miss this stuff."

I handed him the bottle along with a burp cloth and warned him, "She blows sometimes … like Old Faithful. I'm talking explosions!" He assured me that if this happened, he wouldn't be upset.

When we safely landed, this kind man carried Winona and the diaper bag until I was back in the wheelchair that would take me to luggage claim where I'd meet Mom and Dad.

"Thank you *so much* for all your help," I said from the wheelchair, as I held out my arms to take Winona back.

He leaned in and kissed Winona's forehead to tell her goodbye. As he placed her in my arms, all I could think was, *This man saved my day. I don't think I could have flown without him … my saving grace.*

Since that day, I wish I had asked for his name … I wish I had asked for contact information so I could have officially thanked him. I would love to share a picture of Winona today, so many years later, with him. I often wonder if he even recalls that day—his unconditional kindness that saved me so much anxiety. It would be cool to know that he recalls that flight as much as I do. But I have a feeling that he's the type of guy who thought nothing of his help—that maybe he was just thankful for a little baby who helped pass the time on a plane ride. Or, was he an angel? Was he sent to ease my worries, and to help my faith grow when I felt most alone in the world?

I may never know, but I will admit to this … this man was the start of something different in my life. This man helped me in a way I hadn't thought about before—with his kindness and ease that helped lift my fears that day—this man helped me see that even when I thought I was alone, I was not alone.

Getting the Baclofen Pump

"I'M ON BOARD IF YOU THINK I'M A GOOD CANDIDATE FOR this. I am willing to do just about anything at this point. My girls need a mom who is better able to take care of them."

Dr. Fleischer seemed to get it. I was healthy, willing, and had good family support to go through yet another procedure—hopefully a last resort to get my spastic muscles under better control.

Steve went with me that day to meet a neurologist who specialized in intrathecal baclofen pumps. This pump would provide steady dosage of my daily baclofen, and would do it with fewer side effects than my oral baclofen because the medicine would be delivered directly into my spinal column.

I should probably backtrack a little … to when my family physician recommended a new neurologist. Even before my move to Georgia, I had shared my frustrations with Dr. Diaz one day in her office. *Dr. Anderson seems unapproachable to me. But how do I tell Dr. Diaz this without sounding ungrateful for all Dr. Anderson has done for my family and me?*

I did my best to explain that as I matured throughout the past decade—to a woman with a college degree, a career, and hopes for a family someday—Dr. Anderson seemed to be treating the same young girl who he believed should stay close to her parents and be thankful for a good night's sleep.

Dr. Diaz understood. She recommended Dr. Elizabeth French … then both encouraged me to pursue the available treatments to maximize my mobility. Under Dr. French's care, I soon found myself consulting with a neurologist at the Minneapolis Clinic—Dr. Fleischer, who saw the baclofen pump as a viable solution for a spastic mother of two busy little girls.

* * *

Since our move from Georgia, so much had happened. To start with, we were able to bide our time at Mom and Dad's while searching for our own place. Ironically, that first "home" in Minnesota would be the next-door neighbors' basement—a house my parents owned—while my dad built a new house for us in Ramsey. Meanwhile, Steve had experienced a number of job changes, which eventually led to a solid position as a production supervisor. Yet, the career changes stressed us out with months of not knowing. Eventually hired by Entegris, he got stuck with night shifts, while I felt over my head with bedtime baby care for Winona. On top of all of this, I had returned to work for the Social Security Administration.

As Winona matured, some things got easier, while other things made me wonder if I was a good mother. Curious and excited about life, Winona was walking by age one, so I didn't have to carry her around the house. She followed me everywhere I went, with a big grin on her face. She tried to imitate everything I did, including my walk. When I saw her on her tippy-toes, wobbling from room to room, I couldn't help but think, *Does she have it too?* My mom would assure me that she was normal: "You have nothing to worry about." I think that meant that Winona's milestones had far surpassed mine at that same age. Yet the fear of giving spastic diplegia to my child hovered, always.

"I think we should try for another one," Steve stated as he helped me get ready for bed one night.

"What?" I said with horror on my face.

"I think we should have another baby."

My head spun with a million worries. Steve triggered some sort of deep, defensive, survival instinct buried in my psyche. I was so taken aback by this absurd request, I couldn't even respond.

How can he say this? Winona is not even two. I can't lift my own child into her bed at night. I thought I might die almost every day of my last pregnancy.

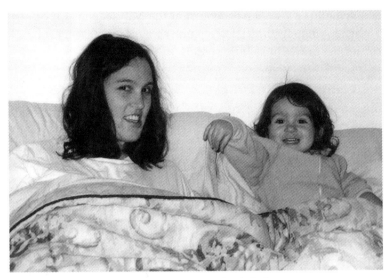

Jean and Winona resting in bed

Who would even consider doing this again? The only reason I entertain the idea of carrying another baby is because the thought of Winona growing up alone, without a sibling for a playmate, makes me profoundly sad.

I closed my eyes to find the strength to speak, yet held back enough so Steve didn't think he had married a monster who only had enough love for one child. "I'm not ready to be pregnant again," I whispered. "I don't know if I can do it."

Steve sat on the edge of the bed and told me all of the good things that would come from having another baby "and giving Winona a friend."

I said what I always did when this topic came up—although it hadn't since Winona was born. "I want to have another child too, but at this moment, I'm just not mentally prepared for the hell it takes for me to grow a baby."

Steve tried another angle. He cozied up a little closer and said that we should try for another one soon so I could "get it over with."

Hmmm... that sounds worse than you meant, honey.

Most people would probably think Steve was digging an even

bigger hole. But, at the time, these were actually the words that got me listening ... the words that got me to consider the thing I dreaded most.

I had always wanted three children, but after delivering my first baby, I knew immediately that I could only endure the stress of pregnancy one more time—and that was mostly because I didn't want Winona to be an only child. That night, Steve made sense to me. *We know that this will take patience and fortitude ... that another horribly difficult pregnancy is inevitable ... so why not just get it over with ...*

A few weeks later, that grumbling, nauseous feeling moved back into my life. My stomach was constantly churning, my breasts were sore, exhaustion crept in slowly. But I knew ... without a doubt, I knew I was pregnant.

A mix of emotions joined the stirring in my stomach. *I am happy that we're going to have another child, but I'm disappointed that it takes nine months of my life to do this.* I felt like I was entered into a marathon against my will, and if I didn't finish, someone would suffer some pretty dire consequences. *This is the last time I have to go through this ... I'll do it for Winona ... I'll do it for Steve ... and for whoever this little brother or sister is.*

Every Monday, my mom picked me up for our evening workout. I always left the gym better than how I arrived. The weights clearly warmed up and stretched out my muscles, just like back in Coach Holland's high school weight lifting class. Afterwards, we would drive to my house and Dad would meet us with a home-cooked meal. My parents stayed for dinner and Winona entertained us all. I loved those Monday nights—even after I realized I was pregnant. I felt so much better with an exercise routine, especially with the workout of a lifetime pending.

This pregnancy was nearly a carbon copy of what I went through with Winona. I knew that my body would never attempt this again, so I talked to the nurse practitioner at my eight-month appointment.

"I want my tubes tied after I deliver," I stated matter-of-factly.

She looked me in the eyes and replied, "You can't make that kind of decision while you're pregnant."

I tried to explain that the decision had been made a long time ago. "I made this decision *between* pregnancies because I knew that I couldn't do this again … and two children are enough for us."

"No, I'm sorry. But that kind of surgery can't be done right after delivery." She tried to get through to me … that this was something I needed to think about *after* I delivered the baby. "You can't be making any drastic decisions while you're pregnant. I mean, it's almost impossible to reverse. You'll need time after this one is born to make sure this is the right thing for you and your family."

Okay, I get it … it's as if we pregnant mothers are not of sound mind … temporary insanity … walking hormone horror shows … weak-minded women who can't make a rational decision while our bellies are bloated and our cankles keep expanding.

Actually, I accepted that.

What I didn't understand was why she couldn't get it through her well-trained mind that this decision was made *after* I had Winona, but *before* my current pregnancy.

I came to this rational decision many months after my daughter was born … I was of sound mind … This is just an interim plan! Can't you respect me for thinking ahead? I am fully content with a family of four. I'm not looking to make a basketball team or a Y2K version of the Partridge Family!

But, her mind was made up and there was nothing I could do about it … thank God!

Despite a similar start to my first trimester, this pregnancy proved to be different than Winona's. I experienced light-headedness that, at first, was quite random. Answering the phone line at work … occasionally on my drive in the morning … but by week thirty-two, it was an almost daily occurrence. On two separate occasions that week, I pulled over just in time to stop from blacking out.

I drank from my water bottle, then reclined my seat all the way back. After about five minutes, the light-headedness passed, so I could finish my drive.

Close to the end of my eighth month, it happened while I was answering the phones. I noticed all of my water was gone, and I knew that I wouldn't make it to the sink for a refill without passing out. Frankly, I could not physically walk anymore without assistance. I took someone's arm everywhere I went … the break room, my car, the bathroom … At this point, all of my co-workers were away from their desks. I considered my options and picked up my phone to call my supervisor.

"Luke, this is Jean. Can you bring me some water? I feel like I'm going to faint."

In less than thirty seconds, he had water in my hands. I drank it quickly, got my bearings, and smiled a thank you, which was Luke's cue that he could go back to his desk.

But the feeling returned—*I'm going to faint.* I tucked my head between my knees and prayed silently that I wouldn't black out. With only one hour left in my workday, I thought I could get through it. *I have to get through it. I have no choice.*

Between head rushes, I called my dad to see if he could pick me up from work. I knew that I couldn't drive home in this condition. It wouldn't be safe for me, my baby, or others on the road.

Marcy walked me out to my dad's car and told me to get some rest. I gave her a weary smile and said, "Goodnight." In my mind, I wasn't sure if I would be back.

Dad drove thirty minutes to get to my work from his house … and brought his friend Gary along to drive my car home. I don't know what I would have done. I have an amazing dad.

Steve took me to see Dr. Carlsen, my obstetrician, the following day.

"I keep feeling faint—like I'm going to pass out," I explained with worry.

He informed me that this was normal and that many women experienced this during pregnancy. But … "You can't drive until after this baby is born."

"What? I have to drive. How will I get to work? Isn't there something you can do?"

"Sorry … I'm afraid not." His smile was a mix of regret and "Deal with it; you're almost done."

I wanted so desperately to work up until the day I delivered, but Dr. Carlsen was not giving me a choice. *My plan was to prove to everyone that I could work through all of this … just like in Georgia. I thought I was so strong ... why do I keep feeling like a failure?* I left the clinic that day depressed since I had to call Luke with my bad news.

Okay—as much as it goes against my grain, I've been given an order to cruise now ... take care of Winona, and wait a few weeks for this baby.

I thought that being home for the rest of my pregnancy would be a piece of cake. I could do light housework at my own pace, take an afternoon snooze while Winona napped, and tend to any final preparations for this new little one. But an unexpected side effect occurred. I experienced vaginal pain that made me question every step before I took it. With a month left to go before being declared full term, I had pain surging through my pelvic bone so severely that I held my crotch with every agonizing step I took. *I can't go anywhere in public ... people will wonder what is wrong with me!*

With two weeks left to go, I was dilated to four centimeters. My mom made me laugh with her favorite line, "If you hear crying, dial 911." I hoped her humor would be only that—a little comic relief.

Baby number two came just like the first ... delivery was almost déjà vu. I was given an epidural, and Pitocin to start labor. *I can't wait to meet this baby and to find out if Winona has a brother or a sister.* I was so grateful that I didn't know the gender, since this became my motivation—a goal to discover ... a detail to fixate on during that day in labor.

Four hours after the beginning stages of labor, Dr. Carlsen announced, "It's time to push." As I pushed, he pulled. Two minutes later, the room filled with cries.

"What is it? A boy or a girl? What is it?" I said, trying to sit up, my legs still locked in place.

No one answered.

"Is it a boy or a girl?" I said more forcefully.

"It's a girl," Dr. Carlsen said calmly. "I thought you already knew."

As the nurse placed my baby girl in my arms, I could see that her big gray eyes and chunky cheeks were perfect! *Sharon Lynn is the final piece to our Abbott puzzle*—a claim I kept for a while.

* * *

Two busy girls, and painful, debilitating spasms ... motherhood brought more than I had bargained for. I was willing to try anything to alter my current course.

"This surgical procedure will put the device inside you—next to your stomach. A catheter will feed the baclofen directly to your cerebral spinal fluid. This will eliminate your need for oral baclofen and all of the side effects that go with high doses of meds over many years." I recall my doctor's explanation, and the feeling of *Bring it on!*

The pump would also direct the baclofen to the targeted area, which would make the medicine much more effective. People who went this route reported feeling stronger, and said they were capable of doing so much more. I wanted this. Especially with my girls growing up so fast—I knew this would improve the quality of our lives if I had more mobility for them. Often, you hear that it is not the health conditions that wear away at people's lives—it is the side effects from all the drugs they use to stay mobile, strong, and alert. So, at the very least, I was optimistic this would help me reduce the amount of medication swimming around in my bloodstream.

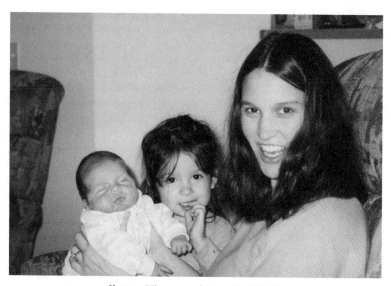

Sharon, Winona, and Jean, April 2004

"You'll need a trial first—a test to see if you'll tolerate baclofen in this way," Dr. Fleischer informed me, with Steve listening too. "You'll have a large dose of baclofen injected into your spine to insure that this works. Having a pump implanted is an invasive procedure—we don't want to put you through it unless you are a good candidate for the pump."

Steve took the day off from work, and we headed to the hospital for the test. My muscles were very spastic and tired since I was instructed to skip my morning meds. I had been taking baclofen for nearly thirty years. My limbs clearly did not understand why they weren't fed the usual 35mg dosage that morning. I was uncomfortable, but hopeful that when I received the injection, my muscles would relax, which would show everyone that the pump was a good option for my disability.

I lay on the firm white medical table and waited for the doctor to come and stick my back with a needle. Slightly chilled by the draft of cool air coming from the vent, I listened to my stomach growl while waiting patiently for the procedure to begin. The thin blue-and-white robe, hospital issue, was not much help. Finally, I heard a knock on the door, and watched a man and a woman, both dressed in blue scrubs, enter the room. They each extended a hand to introduce themselves. *I'm too cold, hungry, and spastic for any socializing. Let's get this show on the road.*

Together, they helped roll me onto my stomach. They were gentle and friendly, and as anxious as I was. I remember appreciating that. Cool air stroked my skin as one of them pulled the gown off of my back. The gentleman spoke first. "I'm going to rub something on the area now, to numb the spot where we will insert the needle." He continued to give me a play-by-play description of everything he was doing. I assumed they must get a lot of nervous people who rarely experienced a hospital stay. I was not that patient. I felt like a pro. *I'm just happy that there will be no surgical cut—only punctures. I won't have to deal with the nausea or grogginess of anesthesia.* I was surprisingly calm and eager to have the trial prove that the baclofen pump was right for me.

A couple minutes after my back received the numbing agent, my skin was sterilized. I was directed to stay completely still. Any movement could increase the chance for paralysis. As difficult as it was for me to walk, I was not about to give my mobility up for good. I did all I could to stay still, but I feared I could not control some of the involuntary movements my body made.

I felt a brief, slight pressure on the base of my spine. The doctor walked toward my head so I could see him. He stared directly into my eyes and said, "Now we wait."

Shortly after the injection, they transferred me to a hospital bed. I finally saw Steve again, once they wheeled me to a room a few floors up. I'm not sure how long he had been waiting there for me, but I found solace in watching him watch the hospital staff lock my bed into place.

"How are you?" he asked.

I tried a smile. It didn't last long.

"I feel sick to my stomach." The nausea couldn't be avoided.

Steve knew—after five years and two pregnancies together, he knew to go to the nurses' station and ask for some crackers. He returned holding a Styrofoam cup in one hand and saltine crackers in the other. Once again he was here to rescue me when I was unable to help myself. He handed me a single cracker, waited for me to eat it, and reached for the cup of water. He put the bent straw between my lips. The ice water moistened my mouth so I could eat another cracker. I took a second sip of water from the cup Steve held, and noticed that expectant look on his face as he waited for my nausea to subside.

A young nurse entered the room and offered to get me something else to eat while I waited for the doctor to examine me. She came back with green Jell-O, which Steve fed to me. My arms were very spastic, but I reminded myself that the shot of baclofen only targeted my legs.

We heard a loud beeping noise from the room next to mine … the sound a garbage truck makes when backing up—only louder. A nurse ran by my room yelling, "Robert, you need to sit down." Steve and I heard her explain to the patient why he needed to stay in his chair. The beeping continued and when it stopped, I assumed that Robert must have finally sat down.

Steve turned on the television. I knew his sudden interest in Maury Povich was simply to drown out the beeping from my elderly neighbor's room. As the host of the show was about to reveal "who the father is," the beeping began again.

BEEP … BEEP … BEEP …

The nurse flew by my room, "Robert, you need to sit down!"

My arms and legs began to spasm almost simultaneously with the beeping and bustle next door. My right hand jolted up to my face, touching my chin. I put it back down by my side, but I couldn't seem to stop clenching my fist. My toes curled toward the bed, cramping the arches of my feet.

BEEP … BEEP … BEEP …

Steve shut the door to my room and returned to the seat next to my bed. The muffled noise of the nurse trying to settle her patient down still captured my attention. The beeping stopped and I made myself take deep breaths in an attempt to control the spasms.

Another hospital bed was abruptly rolled into my room. I watched as a gray-haired woman—I would guess in her seventies—was parked next to me. The hospital staff left the room right after they closed the curtain between the two of us.

Within minutes, my roommate dialed her phone and began shouting to the recipient of her call, obviously a family member. She yelled every response—but mostly the word, "What?"

I don't know if I can take much more of this. All I really want to do is relax until Dr. Fleischer comes to examine me. That's when the beeping began again, along with the spasms in my arms and legs.

BEEP … BEEP … BEEP …

Steve sighed and walked back into the hall. I overheard the nurse explain to Steve that my neighbor had a severe brain injury.

"If he stands up, he could fall and hurt himself even more. But he won't stay put."

Steve then informed her that with every beep, I went into a full-body spasm. I didn't hear everything they said, but within a few minutes, Steve returned to his chair.

An hour later, Dr. Fleischer knocked on my door. He entered the room with a smile and a "Hello." He ran through all of the typical tests that neurologists do, which I've done so many times, I often wonder if I could lead them … *just this once.* Dr. Fleischer moved my legs in several different directions, testing the spasticity level. The rigidity in my legs was definitely worse than normal, and I was suddenly doubtful that the baclofen pump would be the answer to my problems.

Steve spoke up. "She's exhausted and spastic from all of the noise in this room. I don't think it's fair to decide if the pump will work or not when she's fighting all this stress."

Dr. Fleischer apologized and said that he would like to see me walk. His nurse returned with a walker and I sat up on the side of the hospital bed. Dr. Fleischer tied a two-inch-wide white belt around my waist and asked me to stand up using the walker.

"You've got a lot more baclofen in your system than if you had the pump implanted. But this will give me some idea of how you'll do with the pump's steady dose to your spine." Dr. Fleischer encouraged me to stand and take a step.

I grabbed the walker as Steve held onto my side, hoping to keep me balanced. I pushed my bottom off of the bed and stood there for a moment. I looked at Steve's face, searching for optimism to fuel my first steps. He smiled at me and I took a step forward with my left foot.

"Head out of the room and go down the hall," Dr. Fleischer told me.

As I took each step, I felt my right foot drag slightly. This was not normal. I told each of the men at my side that "this is tricky," but I didn't want to give up. I took slow, methodical steps, half expecting Dr. Fleischer to put a stop to this at any moment.

Dr. Fleischer reminded me that, "your muscles received much more baclofen than you would ever need." This would result in noodle-like symptoms—which described my legs to a T. I was holding on to the walker with my strong arms and dragging my spaghetti-noodle legs across the floor. The walk around the loop seemed to take forever. After my marathon lap, I was helped back into my bed, and I wondered who in the room was the true seventy-year-old. I was convinced that the trial had failed.

I am not a good candidate for the pump. My hopes of having a better gait and taking less medication are out the window. Please, Lord, I want to be a more involved mother. There's got to be a way to make this work! But just as fast as my hopes faded, Dr. Fleischer informed me that the trial went really well. He told Steve, "She's a good candidate for the baclofen pump." He told me, "Let's get you recovered from this procedure and ready for the next step."

I wondered if we witnessed the same results that day. Had my doctor been talking to me, but watching someone else take confident laps around the hospital hallway? Of course, I wanted to trust Dr. Fleischer—I needed to believe that despite my struggle that morning, the real medical device, the actual pump, would have much better results.

Steve and I agreed—I would give this a try … although this was not exactly a new sofa we could return to Slumberland if we discovered it did not match our décor after all.

Actually, we both knew better. This surgery was not going to be easy for either of us. But having the hockey puck device under my skin—with tubing winding internally toward and up my spine—I might see baclofen as a normal part of my body chemistry. It would fix nature … my nature that had been messed with since birth.

Dr. Fleischer gave his final blessing, and warned me about the recovery time.

"You'll need to keep calm and flat while the hole in your spine closes. No baby care for a while."

If it worked—if it led to a less spastic future for me and my kids, it would be a short-lived trade-off. *I have been through much worse in my day. This should be just another adventure to add to my list. With Steve, my parents, and God by my side, I will get through this. No problem!*

Pump Woes

I AWOKE TO THE FAMILIAR SILENCE OF A HOSPITAL ROOM, comfortably numb in the Minneapolis hospital bed. Gray, sterile walls blended in with the cloudy haze outside my window. A dull silence amplified my loneliness. *At least the pain medication is doing its job.* Even before the first nursing shift change of the day, Steve and my parents arrived by my bedside with reassuring smiles and pats to my shoulder and legs.

The three of them had been my saving grace and always will be. In those early years of marriage, Steve, my rock, would endure so much more than most husbands and wives had to experience in a lifetime together. My parents, the other force behind me, made me wonder what kind of person I would have been without their dedication and constant love. They respected my marriage, playing a quiet but supportive role when things were normal—at least my normal. But in a medical crisis, Steve and I knew they would be present … they would know exactly what to do and how to help.

Now that my pump was in place, Steve needed to go to work. Mom sat by my side throughout the two hospital recovery days. She was there to pass the time, to laugh with me at people on TV, and to hold the barf bowl after the pain medication got the best of me.

"No more pain killers," I said, as Mom wiped my mouth with a damp cloth. "They're making me sick again." As a little girl, I would always vomit after surgeries. My stomach just can't handle the poison that drips from an IV.

"I'd rather feel horrible pain than puke." I said to my mom with my eyes welling up.

"I know," she said, wiping the hair from my face.

The afternoon nurse arrived and informed me that it had been twenty-four hours. "It's time to sit up." She slowly raised the back of the bed to a sitting position and informed me that if this didn't produce a headache, I would be expected to get out of the bed and sit in the recliner. This was music to my ears. I knew the drill. The sooner I got out of bed, the sooner I could go home. I hated being in the hospital and I feeling like I would never recover. There was just something about being home that relaxed my muscles and my mind.

Luckily, I had no headache, so the nurse came to my side to help me to the chair. Slowly and cautiously, I swung my legs off the right side of the bed. My mom stood on one side of me and the nurse stood on the other. They each took an arm. As I scooched to the edge of the bed, the pain seared through the bottom right side of my back. *What is that? I know I have an incision on my stomach, but why does my back hurt like someone is twisting a hot poker right through me?*

I looked at the nurse. "It hurts too bad to move."

"I'll go get me more pain medication."

"No!" I quickly replied. "That will make me sick."

She urged me to take the medication, but I insisted that I would get out of this bed without it. *I will not take more of the drugs that make me vomit!*

I asked for a few minutes ... to get my mind ready for the pain. *I can do this. I know I can. I have been through much worse than this.*

Mom took a seat in the recliner, showing patience while I prepared for the painful move. Meanwhile, a frail, gray-haired woman knocked on the open hospital-room door. "The hospital records show that you are Catholic. Would you like me to give you Communion?" She showed me the small golden case she was holding.

"Sure." Although I could not physically stand up to accept the round, flat host, the woman came in close to me.

"The Body of Christ." I made the sign of the cross just as I did every Sunday as a child growing up.

"Do you have a special prayer that you prefer to say?" she asked Mom and me.

I had no words, but my mother was quick to ask for a prayer to help lessen my pain so I could get to the chair. I was grateful for Mom's request, but my thoughts slipped into my usual pattern ...

There are greater needs in the world. People are homeless; children are dying of cancer; patients are being airlifted to this hospital every day ... and we ask for help getting me to a chair? Well, if God thinks I am worthy ... I didn't have the strength to object. I closed my eyes as the little old lady prayed for me.

The nurse returned. "It's time to try again."

My mom and the nurse teamed up for another try. Again, they coaxed my legs to the side of the bed. I forced myself to a sitting position, keeping my back straight. *If I don't lean forward when I stand, the pain will be more tolerable.* I took my mom's arm and the nurse's arm for balanced support. I slowly pushed my feet against the floor and raised my butt off the safety of the bed. I was standing!

The two women continued to hold me as I took two steps to the chair. Gracefully, I turned my body to the left and, with the assistance of my two trusted guides, I slowly lowered myself into the recliner where Mom had been sitting for nearly a day. As soon as my butt and back touched the chair, I knew that I had succeeded. Suddenly, I realized something completely unexpected—it didn't even hurt. *Did the nurse put drugs in my IV without me knowing? Or had God answered our prayers?*

* * *

I missed my girls throughout the hospital stay, but had been thankful that their routine was pretty closely followed, despite my absence. They went to daycare as usual while I underwent my baclofen pump procedure. For some time, we had been paying a neighbor lady to babysit within her home. She had no children, and seemed willing to come to our door to get the girls, walk them to her own house, then return them once she spotted my car pulling in each afternoon around 4:30 P.M. Steve was working long second shifts, and since I could never load up two children into a car to haul them to a center, the neighborhood daycare was a viable solution.

After a few more days at home to recoup, I was back to work three days a week. Hidden under my clothing, a six-inch elastic band around my waist held the hockey puck-sized pump in place as prescribed. My co-workers were supportive and welcoming with comments like, "I think your walking has improved … for sure … I agree."

I straightened my posture with their words and was so grateful for the slight improvement in my gait. I felt more independent at work. I could reach the break room on my own and stride to the copier without feeling like the ground was shaking beneath me.

At home, I noticed big changes, too. Prior to the pump, I wasn't able to turn my body to the right while walking. For instance, when I would walk to the bathroom from my bedroom, I would walk to the door, stop, then turn left in a three-quarter circle (270 degrees) in order to enter the bathroom. After the pump, at least in those first few days home from the hospital, I finally took a right turn. In addition, my furniture walking—my hands on the back of the sofa … step, step … to the arm of a nearby chair for balance … step, step … to the closest kitchen chair—also ended. *The pump is the answer I have been looking for my whole life.*

* * *

My post-surgery honeymoon ended gradually. It seemed to start with normal itchy stitches, but eventually my life spun out of control.

After a few days of healthy healing, it took everything in my power not to scratch the surgical site and rip open my stitches. During the day, I resisted, but when I finally crawled into bed at night, my hands would attack. The neurologist told me to "take Benadryl … it should go away."

After three days back at work, I couldn't tolerate the itch any longer. To make matters worse, my chest had the same sensation. I contacted the neurosurgeon's nurse and she prescribed an antibiotic.

"Start it as soon as you can pick it up, but if you come down with a fever, go to the ER immediately." I put in a leave slip and headed home to find my parents there, offering to pick up the prescription. Dad left and returned from the pharmacy so fast, I hardly knew he was gone.

"Mom, my whole body is itchy now!" I cried. "Even my legs."

My mom saw the weakness in my body, agreed to watch the girls, and helped me to bed. She handed me a glass of water so I could swallow the pill that Dad had delivered in record time. After two doses of the medication and a good night's sleep, the itching finally subsided. On the phone the next day, the surgeon insisted this was not a staph infection, while my neurologist was confident it was.

I continued to see Dr. Fleischer on a monthly basis so he could increase my baclofen pump dosage and reduce the oral baclofen. With each successive appointment, my walking worsened. Every day, I became more apprehensive about walks to the mailbox or the bathroom at work. Eventually, the walk from my car into work became a new fear—something that had never been an issue before since the mornings were always my best times. My legs lost so much stability that I started to doubt their capacity to hold me up. As my confident posture and gait faded, my anxiety about leaving the house increased.

Dr. Fleischer increased my pump-fed baclofen again, yet I felt my limbs grow progressively unstable.

"I'm nervous to go anywhere by myself."

Dr. Fleischer informed me that he was unsure if he should raise or decrease the amount of baclofen in my pump. "What do you want me to do?" he asked with concern.

"I don't know," I said with tears filling my eyes.

"I'm going to have you increase your diazepam," he stated. I had previously taken this drug—which most people know as Valium— for spasms, but it is more commonly used for anxiety.

I was in no shape to argue. I accepted this new dosage, and left with a medication to help my mind adjust to what was happening to my body. But clearly no plan was in place to help my body correct the issue at hand.

In retrospect, I wonder why Dr. Fleischer didn't seem to be questioning whether the pump was working at all. *Would he get to a point where he would admit that I simply was not a good candidate for the pump? That maybe I was destined to take oral baclofen my whole life? Should I pray for something new and better to come along?* Oddly, none of these questions crossed my lips in our monthly meetings. *Was my desire to have the pump work overpowering my judgment to question what was best for my health?*

Things at work got worse. I couldn't walk anywhere on my own. I couldn't even think about trying to get to the bathroom to pee. I would stop there each morning just before I trudged to my desk for a full day. I held my urine from 8:55 A.M. until I arrived home at 4:30 P.M. To avoid the sensation that my bladder might burst, I drank little to nothing all day long. I felt yucky most of the afternoon from dehydration. Still, by the time I reached my house, I never knew if I would wet my pants before I got to the toilet.

To make matters worse, our daycare neighbor seemed put out when I requested that she keep the girls until 5:30 every day.

"But I can see you're coming home at 4:30. Don't you want to see your girls right away?"

"I know they are probably ready to be home with me, but if I just take a nap for that hour after work, I'll have the stamina to deal with them through dinner and bedtime." This seemed so rational to me, but I could tell this woman was beginning to judge me as a deadbeat mother. She knew of another arrangement I had with one very kind and generous neighbor who brought dinner to us one evening per week.

This ambitious mother of ten barely agreed to the few dollars we gave her for the ingredients—"If I cook for twelve or fourteen, what's the difference? You and your girls eat like birds compared to my big eaters. But if you insist, you can only pay me for the portion of groceries." One of her kids delivered the meal, and Steve was sometimes lucky enough to get a few leftovers. This meal, a few peanut butter and jelly nights, and one meal per week from Mom got us through until Steve could cook on the weekends.

Feeling less than Mother-of-the-Year, along with added stress at work as I covered up for my decline in mobility, I wondered how long I could continue at this pace. As Steve helped me pull down my pants day after day when I got home from work, he always asked, "Why don't you use the bathroom right before you leave?" One day, I finally told him that I couldn't make it there on my own anymore. This seemed to surprise him. He wasn't angry with me, but he now understood how far the pump situation had gone ... far enough to deem it a failure.

I called Dr. Fleischer's office to request that they "shut the thing off."

"It needs to be decreased little by little," the nurse informed me. "There's a risk of death if we stop it abruptly." I made the appointment to start the process.

Steve joined me at this appointment. Through our discussion, the doctor learned of my struggles at work. The bathroom stunt seemed to be the final straw. "You cannot return to work," the doctor stated firmly. Steve showed relief at this statement. Of course, my health was at risk and they were looking out for me, but I felt betrayed—as if two grown men were taking my rights away, and grounding me to my room.

Work had always been important to me. A job made me feel worthy ... that I wasn't a burden to society, but instead a contributor. *I'm not going to have that taken away from me.* The anger and sadness overwhelmed me as I realized I was outnumbered and too weak to fight the battle. Speechless, I left the clinic with Steve, who practically carried me to the car.

"Do you want to stop at work on the way home to get your things?" Steve asked.

"I can't face any of them," I said, staring out the window.

For the first time in my life, I had nothing to say. Thoughts of my days at the Social Security office swirled around in my mind. My first day on the job ... the showers given by co-workers for my wedding and babies ... my friendly rapport with so many new clients. I once helped a woman who was suicidal on the phone. Because of me, she got help and no longer felt like the government was "out to get her."

Then there was my award in 2006 that made me realize I had supervisors who acknowledged and respected my hard work ethic … that they could see I did my job well, despite my disability.

Our selection for 2006 Civil Servant of the Year is Jean Abbott. We believe that Jean's excellent interpersonal and customer service skills make her an excellent choice for Civil Servant of the Year. Jean is an empathetic interviewer and has a real flair for establishing an amicable rapport between herself and the public. Her great attitude goes a long way toward strengthening the partnership between the public and our office. Jean always goes the "extra mile" for each person with whom she comes in contact.

Please join us in congratulating her on this honor. The awards luncheon will be held Friday, May 5, 2006, at the Sheraton Hotel in Bloomington. We will send out details about the luncheon when we receive it from FEB, for those of you who are interested in attending.

Veronica, Kenneth, and Mia

Just when others see that I do make a difference, I have to quit? If I don't have work, what do I have?

Obviously, my life was full of so many blessings, with Steve, our kids, and a loving extended family. Yet, at that moment, I couldn't see the good in it. I only felt loss—as if I had been robbed or violated of personal possessions. I had always been one to love my life. Even with all of my physical issues, it was my nature to see the good in life's challenges. *So, why can't I stop crying? I'm home with my beautiful, fun-loving daughters, yet I wake up sad and go to bed sad, and feel cheated because I can't work like a normal person.* My inability to use the bathroom or take a shower or go to the store without assistance from my mom or Steve magnified my new negative outlook. My antidote: tears.

After a week of crying off and on all day, every day, I finally spoke up for myself. I told my mom and Steve that I needed to see a counselor, and Mom, once again, graciously offered to take me there, for what became weeks of talk therapy.

Kate, a very caring listener, heard me express my deepest thoughts about living with spastic diplegia. "Depression and anxiety are paralyzing me … and it's far worse than anything physical that my disability has ever forced me to deal with."

She provided the empathy I needed, then informed me, "You are essentially dealing with a death. Being told that you can no longer work—facing this level of loss of mobility and independence—it's very similar to having a spouse or a parent die."

I looked at her and wondered, *Is she overstating it? I've never lost a parent or a spouse, but if I did, I think this is how it would feel. I eat, breathe, and sleep the loss of what little mobility I had … of going backwards. I can't do anything on my own anymore, even in my own home.* I was so relieved to find one person who understood how huge this was … *Thank God, someone gets it.*

At night, I relied on Winona to put me to bed. She was five years

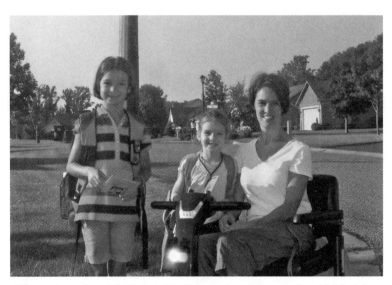

Winona (second grade), Sharon (kindergarten), and Jean on the girls' first day of school

221

old. *I should still be tucking her into bed at night. This is so reversed—it's so wrong.* Like a hired caregiver, Winona helped me into my pajamas and then into bed. I felt as if I was robbing her of her childhood. She genuinely loved being by my side. She was always happy to help me. But many nights I fought the melancholy that came as she made peanut butter and jelly sandwiches for me, Sharon, and herself, which we ate in my bedroom once I was securely in bed. I ate lying down while the girls sat on a bath towel, chewing away as if we were at the beach ... but instead of a view of the lake, we watched a tape of Curious George and his silly antics. Apparently, the girls really enjoyed this. On the days when the kind neighbor brought over our dinner, they asked if we could "eat it in the bedroom on our towels?"

After two months of spilling my heart out to Kate, I felt better and more accepting of the loss of my job. *Maybe not working is what I need. I can have more quality time with the girls ... and take a nap every day so I can refuel for the evening.* I wanted to get back to making dinners, even if I had to prepare them in the morning for reheating at 5:00 P.M.

On my last visit, I thanked Kate. "You've saved my life. I'm ready for a new way of looking at things—I couldn't have done this without your help."

* * *

Dr. Fleischer had been increasing and decreasing my baclofen dosage, which put me officially at my worst. Physically, I could hardly sit up on my own because of the amount of medication in my system. The only way I could sit was if I had armrests on each side of me. Sitting was something I had never had a problem with, so this was evidence that I had become measurably worse. Both my parents and Steve told me, "It's time for a second opinion."

My mom said that she would take me to another neurologist.

"I can't tell my story to one more person. I don't have the strength."

"I can do it for you ... I will do all of the talking. I can make the appointment, drive you there, and do all the health history." I agreed and Mom called the rehabilitation center that specialized in baclofen pumps.

During my next appointment, I told Dr. Fleischer that I had a plan to see another doctor ... "I need my records sent to The Courage Center."

He told me not to be surprised if they couldn't help me.

Good Friday

WE PULLED INTO THE PARKING LOT OF THE LOCAL REHABILI-
tation center, and Mom walked around to my side of the car to help
me out. I clutched her arm and focused on each and every step I
took until I could safely sit in a waiting-room chair. We patiently
anticipated my name to be called.

Dr. Griffith entered the examination room smiling, and greeted
me with, "Hello," followed by a familiar look … she appeared ready
to hear my story. My eyes met my mom's … her cue to start sharing
what I didn't have the energy to express for the umpteenth time.

I listened and observed. Dr. Griffith gave a much different first
impression than the doctors I had seen over the past three decades.
She listened intently, without passing judgment. She looked concerned. I thought to myself, *For once, we've met a doctor who isn't going
to put words in my mouth.* After listening to my mom talk for over
thirty minutes, Dr. Griffith asked to examine me.

"Sounds to me like you are being over medicated with baclofen
and it probably needs to be reduced," she stated matter-of-factly. She
also stated that she was a bit confused about my diagnosis. "What
is it?"

"Spastic diplegia," I finally spoke for myself in my strongest
whisper.

She perused my records from Dr. Fleischer's office and informed
me of a report that he wrote. "He says right here that your disability
is degenerative and that it's not spastic diplegia."

With wide-eyed fury I replied, "He never told me that!"

Dr. Griffith suggested that in addition to decreasing my baclofen every week, I should consult with a colleague of hers to get a second opinion. "She's a great neurologist."

Finally, Dr. Griffith concurred with Dr. Fleischer's report … "Your diagnosis of spastic diplegia could be incorrect. A good deal of research has been documented since you were diagnosed with this in the early 80s."

I told her, "I was seen by the best as a child … all along, actually. I also went to one of the top hospitals in the United States. I've seen dozens of neurologists over the years and there was never a question regarding my diagnosis." I paused, but stated frankly, "I just want to get my baclofen pump regulated to a proper dosage." She looked at me with understanding and told me to let her know if and when I wanted the information to meet the other neurologist.

Over the next few months, I visited Dr. Griffith weekly, then biweekly, and finally monthly, until my pump was reduced to nothing. In that time, the degree of controlled spasticity required for daily function returned to me. I could sit in a chair; I started using the bathroom on my own; I could walk from room to room within my own house again. I wasn't at my optimum self, but things progressed faster than I expected. *I thought I'd be in a wheelchair full time by now—this is far better than where I was headed.*

At the next appointment, I thanked Dr. Griffith for all her help—for giving me so much attention and really listening to what my mom and I had to say. Then I asked for her friend's contact information.

"The neurologist you thought I should see? Is that offer still good?"

She smiled and grabbed a pad of paper. She wrote the name Stephanie Williams followed by a phone number on the top sheet before tearing it off for me.

I informed Dr. Griffith that contacting her recommended neurologist was "the least I could do considering how much you have helped me."

"Good. But don't do it for me. Do it for yourself. I think you will be surprised at how she can help you." I thanked Dr. Griffith and left the clinic feeling indifferent but obligated to try the phone number she shared with me.

Thankfully, turning the baclofen pump off brought some degree of drive back to my role as Mom. Over time, I had come to fully accept that being a physically challenged mother was harder than I had anticipated. Beyond the physical hardship of not being able to lift my own kids off the ground if they fell, I felt the sting of the emotional inadequacy that grew with every limitation I faced. For instance, other parents simply hopped in the car to run their kids to activities. In fact, I sometimes overheard them complaining about the "running" they had to do if their child was in soccer or Girl Scouts. I, on the other hand, spent my energy coordinating rides from other parents for Winona who had already reached the age of joining teams and activities. Sharon would be doing the same thing in no time, and I already worried about coordinating another set of car pools in which I could not participate. Hauling the girls around in the car would have been a breeze compared to swallowing my pride and asking someone to basically be our taxi service.

In retrospect, I am so grateful for those who said yes, and fully understand why people were so willing to help. I love it when a busy mom calls me up and asks for help with her child now that I can do the running! Yet, during those difficult days when my need for support with Winona and Sharon was a direct byproduct of my disability, I truly hated to ask. I only did it because I knew our kids should not pay a price for my stubbornness. *Why should my limitations dictate Winona's experiences?* I had to learn to accept this style of parenting so my kids had opportunities to do what I did growing up. *My parents made so many sacrifices for me growing up ... mine are different, but it's definitely my turn.*

* * *

Meanwhile, my appointment to see Dr. Stephanie Williams arrived on the calendar. I had told my story to so many neurologists over the years; I truly dreaded this new commitment and felt it was point-less. I had gone downhill so fast between the ages of thirty and thirty-three. I had become dependent on everyone. Yet, if Steve and my brother Mike were willing to take time off from work to get me to hear one more opinion, it was best to just go along for the ride.

Mike picked me up at Mom's house and drove me an hour to Dr. Williams's clinic in St. Louis Park. We had planned on eating lunch along the way, but due to poor directions, we ran too late to go through even a drive-up window. Exhausted, hungry, and shaky, I knew my arms and legs were far too spastic to walk from the park-ing ramp to the office. So, Mike grabbed a wheelchair by the sliding doors that connected the parking garage to the hospital. Once he helped me into the chair, he raced me up to the fourth floor, where we were greeted by Steve. He had been waiting for us, ready to guide me back to the clinic room where my life would change forever.

Dr. Williams greeted us and I apologized for being overly spastic and trembling. She listened to the three of us for the most important forty-five minutes of my life. I spoke little since I was so uncomfort-able and knew that Steve could explain my situation as well as me, if not better.

"It's like someone pressed a reset button after she sleeps all night or takes a nap," Steve explained to Dr. Williams.

Her face lit up with an excitement that I had never seen in a doctor before. "What if I told you that there's a pill for you to take that will change the way you walk. From this … " she said as she stood up and started imitating my walk, "to this." She changed her walk drastically. She went from the Hunchback of Notre Dame to the newly crowned Miss America.

Dr. Williams sat down and explained, "I am almost certain you have dopa-responsive dystonia." She explained that my brain didn't make enough dopamine. "You should begin taking Sinemet—a medication typically given to Parkinson's patients." She wrote the prescription out and gave it to Steve and that was it. If Steve hadn't been at this appointment, I wouldn't have filled the prescription and kept thinking, *This doctor is crazy!* I've taken many medications, had years of physical therapy and surgeries, how can one little pill change my life this drastically?

When Steve and I got home, he asked me if I had taken the new medication.

"No, I'll start it tomorrow," I explained, without adding my inner doubts. *Why bother? Dr. Anderson would have prescribed this medication if it was truly important enough to make a difference.*

But Steve insisted. He even buttered me a piece of bread to eat with it, since the bottle of medication clearly stated "take with food." I did as he suggested, taking the first little yellow pill, expecting nothing to change.

And then it started ... although I admit, I did not attribute these early changes to the medication. Call me stubborn ... or just clueless. I had taken the medication for over twenty-four hours and indeed noticed a change in my mobility. My arms were allowing me to move more freely and my legs listened. For the first time in months, or was it years, my brain directed traffic and every one of my limbs followed directions without dispute. I chalked it up to better sleep that night ... until the holiday weekend told me differently.

It was Easter morning, and I got out of bed, braced for a long, physically hard day. I had stayed up late the night before, preparing and hiding the girls' Easter baskets—hard work for me, but a project I enjoyed. Then, for some reason, I barely slept. I tossed and turned, and could not fall into the deep REM sleep my disability craved. I awoke the next morning knowing I would battle my own body all day long.

Holidays were always stressful for me, and a holiday without sleep the night before felt like a curse, not a happy occasion. Easter morning would be filled with the hustle and bustle of the girls searching for their Easter baskets, followed by the challenge of slowing them down long enough to get their frilly dresses on and their hair combed. My hands usually struggled to stop shaking long enough to place hair bands around their pigtails, only to find their father ripping them out and redoing my sloppy attempts.

This particular Easter morning was different. I slowly got out of bed, anticipating a spastic reaction that would keep me from

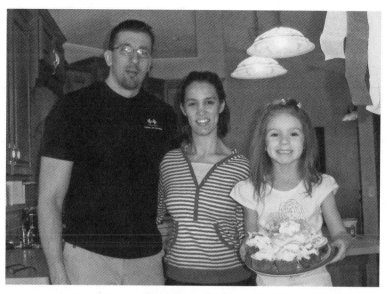

Steve, Jean, and Sharon on Sharon's sixth birthday

showering independently. But then I stood—I stepped from my bed, and, oddly, felt almost strong. I walked to the shower and turned the water on until it was the warm temperature that I preferred. I sidestepped onto the ceramic tile. I let the water hit my body, so as not to get my hair wet because it had been nearly three years since I had last washed my hair alone. But suddenly I reached my arms and hands up and felt the water run through my hair. I had commanded my hands to the top of my head and I was rinsing my hair as my arms cooperated. To me, this was the equivalent of someone picking up the violin after years of not playing to discover they hadn't lost one ounce of talent. It was a familiar feeling, but foreign since it had been so long since I had washed my hair by myself.

I waited for the bomb to drop: For the moment I would have to call out for Steve to "come here and help me out of the shower," as I had done so many times. But it didn't happen. Something had changed. I didn't need his help. Yet, I still didn't want to believe it—I was waiting for this ease in my movement to pass as it always had on those minor occasions when I thought I was better.

Steve and I watched the girls search for their baskets. Then we made our way to the car for our drive to morning mass.

Mass at St. Patrick's is always followed by an Easter egg hunt. The children run out the back doors of church to hunt for plastic Easter eggs. Steve walked with me and the girls into the cool air to meet Sophia, Jack, and Henry, all first cousins, for the colorful egg hunt.

"I'll be right back," Steve said, leaving me on the cement sidewalk that led to the church cemetery.

Panic flashed in my mind. *I don't know if I can stand here by myself with nothing to hold on to.* I didn't have my mom, sister-in-law, brother, father, or even one of the girls to grab onto if I lost my balance. Options raced through my mind. *Should I walk back to the church? No, I'll never make it. Am I going to fall? I'm not sure. What's my landing spot if I do? The sidewalk? The grass?*

Strangely, I seemed to be holding my own.

I'm doing it. I'm standing by myself. I didn't feel off balance, or weak, or even tired after that sleepless night.

It was Easter morning and I was standing alone for the first time in years! I became ever so calm and patient and confident. It was as though Jesus Christ had risen from the dead and he was standing there with me, preparing me to start my new life.

My mom walked toward me with a smile on her face. "I didn't see you," she explained. "I didn't know that it was you standing over here all by yourself!" ... as if she didn't recognize me ... as if I looked different ... maybe stronger, more confident.

It was at that moment—that look of pure relief on my mother's face—when I realized a miracle had happened. It wasn't a coincidence that I was diagnosed on Good Friday, then discovered that my new medication worked on Easter Sunday. The Lord had been with me on this entire journey. He never left my side. He knew I had succumbed to doubt—that I had become so weak in my faith after the baclofen pump debacle—I wouldn't see how important this moment of healing was unless I connected it to the celebration of His son ... to Jesus Christ's Resurrection.

Clarity came with sudden and welcomed force.

Good Friday! It had been Good Friday when Mike wheeled me in to see Dr. Williams—just three days ago when she diagnosed me with something new but treatable. I had this incredibly clear memory of her handing Steve my new prescription. It was close to three o'clock … Friday afternoon. Our church, as well as many secular historians, believe that Jesus died on the cross at that same hour. *This isn't a coincidence.*

At that moment, standing strong and watching my girls run around the backyard of our church, I felt my faith return. It was never really gone—just hiding behind all of the pain of my condition. *How could I see it any other way? This is a miracle.* This was a profound moment for me as my weakened faith suddenly allowed me to see things with a clear and humble mind. *Jesus died for us on the cross … He sacrificed everything for us. And now God has given me a new outlook on life. He's showing me I had the gift of a life worth living all along.*

After that day—that memorable Easter Sunday—I vowed I would no longer say that I'm struggling because of a lack of sleep the night before. I still have restless nights from time to time, and my current doctor reminds me that dopa-responsive dystonia is sleep-sensitive. In fact, I sometimes fight the internal freak-out that this new diagnosis is a mistake … a dream that will be taken away. This invariably happens when I am on a sleepless stretch—a demanding trend of time where I am trying to do too much with little rest. Physical stress definitely influences my disorder, and despite the magic pill that Dr. Williams prescribes, I must nourish my body with breaks, a full night's sleep, and stress-free thoughts as well.

Yet, even when I am tired, I am awed by the fact that my brain can send messages through my nervous system to allow me to walk, to chop food with a sharp knife, to hold a book if I want to read, and to lift my baby from his crib. I don't know of anyone else who lived the first thirty-three years of life crippled, then discovered the opportunity to grasp life in such a new and different way. What a gift … to realize that the little things in our daily experiences make our time here so meaningful and important.

One week later.

I closed the door behind me, leaving six-year-old Sharon alone in the house long enough for me to step out for the mail. I grabbed the rail and descended the seven steps that led to my scooter at the base of the garage stairs. I pressed the button and gradually watched as the garage door slowly opened to reveal the mailbox at the end of my driveway.

I stood there for a brief moment asking myself if I should walk the short distance rather than use my scooter. I took a deep breath, then slid onto the scooter seat. *Maybe tomorrow.*

I drove the scooter to the end of the driveway, stopping at the metal mailbox that read 5730. I peeked inside to find that I was too early. *No mail.* I maneuvered my scooter wheels around and headed back up the driveway. Suddenly, a sheet of notebook paper on the front lawn, and a desire to recover it before it blew away, captured my attention.

I looked to my left and then to my right. No one was around to witness me taking my first steps out there in the wide-open space of our lawn. *This is good … my luck I'll fall to my knees and a neighbor will come racing out after me.*

I motored a little farther up the driveway. As long as the coast was clear, I could park my scooter and retrieve the litter. I looked again to see if any neighbors had come outside, or if any cars were nearing from a distance. *All clear.*

I swung my legs to the right and stepped off the scooter. After a deep breath, I slowly walked the ten steps to where the paper fluttered on the lawn. Before I leaned over to pick it up, I looked again to see that no one was within observation distance.

As I straightened up, I noticed another piece of litter not more than fifteen steps away.

I glanced again at my deserted road, then strode to the stranded trash that had blown to one side of our yard. I walked along the side of my house, to a spot where my feet had never stood, even though I had lived there for seven years. I approached the plastic water bottle on the lawn, bent down, and picked it up.

I could see the neighbor's yard, adjacent to my own back yard, and spotted yet another piece of paper that had blown to the back of our house. My legs carried me down the steep part of our yard, where I picked up that paper too.

The blue swing set where my girls played day after day sat just outside our basement patio door. I spied another plastic water bottle resting a couple of feet away from the slide. I walked to the bottle, reached down, and picked it up.

I should continue in the direction that I am going rather than turn around and go back, I thought after I realized I now had walked more than halfway around my house. I headed up the steep hill on the other side of my house, taking one slow step at a time, leaning forward about thirty degrees to help balance my body up the hill. About fifteen steps later, I had made it to the top and I was standing next to the trash near our garage. I was relieved that the next-door neighbors had not seen this.

I lifted the garbage can lid, which revealed a stench from last week's leftovers. I quickly threw my armful of trash into the can, then turned to face my scooter. I stood completely upright, all by myself. I looked up at the sky and reveled in the warm sun as I smiled at one of my greatest accomplishments to date. *Thank you, Lord, for giving me the capacity to walk around the outside of my house for the first time ever, all by myself.*

I got on my scooter, motored forward, and parked it in the garage. I hopped off, walked up the stairs that led into the house, then spotted Sharon standing in the kitchen, evidently waiting for me.

"I'm sorry that took so long," I smiled. "I ended up walking around the house to pick up garbage that had blown into our yard."

Sharon looked up at me with her big hazel eyes. Tears began rolling down her cheeks.

"What is it, Sharon?" I asked her frantically. "Did you think I had left? I would never leave you," I said, taking a seat at the kitchen table and motioning for her to come sit on my lap.

She walked toward me and looked in my eyes. "No, I'm just so happy." Sharon stopped crying long enough to inform me, "I can't believe you walked outside … without your scooter. I can't believe it, Mommy."

Highlights While Healing

IN ORDER TO HAVE MORE FAMILY TIME, STEVE AND I MOVED our family closer to downtown and Steve's work. The trees outside my condo windows were bare and motionless. It was about 12:30 in the afternoon and it was only Sharon and me at home. What a great day for Halloween. The weather was unseasonably warm and there was no rain or snow in the forecast for trick-or-treating.

Sharon ran to my bedroom and grabbed the clown makeup, big red nose, and rainbow-striped wig from my dresser, then met me in her bathroom. She handed me the tiny rubber band and a black brush that looked like it might belong to a cat. I smiled at Sharon and gently turned her body so she was facing away from me. I brushed her sandy blonde hair and put it into a ponytail. Then I pulled her hair almost all the way through the band one more time, but stopped so it stayed up in what I called a "sloppy bun."

"Here," I said as I patted the edge of the tub—my signal for her to sit down. "I want you to sit here while I put the makeup on you."

I took a seat on the closed toilet and turned sideways so I could face my six-year-old daughter. Her eyes were big with excitement as she sat wearing her pink-and-white sparkling jeans and her cherry-red panda bear shirt with ruffles around the neck that said, "Love" in black letters. I was equally excited to be sitting with her, knowing that this was the first Halloween that I would be able to walk from house to house without the nervousness of growing tired too quickly, or the fear of tripping on the sidewalk.

"What do you want your makeup to look like?" I asked.

"I don't know," Sharon replied.

"Well, do you want to be a happy clown or a sad one?" I asked her patiently.

"Happy!" she said with a bright smile.

"Okay. I need you to be very still, because I don't want the makeup to smudge or go into your eyes. If it goes into your eyes, it could sting, kinda like soap does when you take bath."

I bent down and threw the black-and-white shagged bathmat to the side to prevent getting makeup on it. I did not take this moment for granted knowing that just two years ago I was not able to sit in a chair without being propped up to prevent me from falling over. I took a paper towel and placed it on my lap so I would have somewhere to set the clown makeup. I opened the box of colors. It looked like five short crayons wrapped in gold paper rather than makeup. I took the red crayon with my right hand and placed my left hand on top of Sharon's head.

I drew a line going all the way around her mouth, forming a

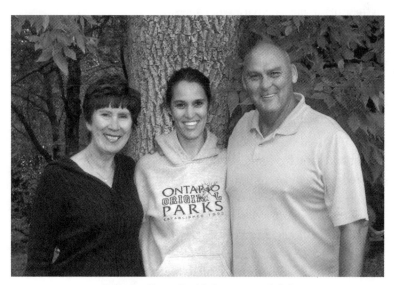

Jean standing tall with her mom and dad

large smile. I felt the miracle of a steady hand at work. *I think she may actually look like a clown by the time I'm done.* I placed the red crayon back into the package and grabbed the green one. I began to draw a dot on the center of her forehead.

"No," Sharon said. "I want red dots."

I explained to her that I had already made the first dot green "and I can't change it now." I could see the wheels turning in her head. She was fine with whatever I did to her face. Her bright eyes told me that she was just happy that my hands were not only capable of holding a colored pencil, but that I was able to color on her face without the frustration of making a mess.

"Okay," she said. "You can do any colored dots, but I want red cheeks."

"I can do that," I said, setting down the green and grabbing for the red again. I outlined a red circle just a little bit bigger than a quarter on her right cheek and then did it again on her left cheek. Again, I colored in the circle perfectly within the lines that I'd created. "This looks good," I told Sharon.

"I wanna see!" she said as she jumped up and took a quick peek in the mirror, pleased with what she saw.

"All right, sit back down so I can finish you up."

Sharon hurried back over to her spot on the tub. I continued to make green circles and added a few blue ones to her face. I finished by drawing blue circles around the outside of her eyes, connecting them over the bridge of her nose, making the appearance of glasses.

Sharon walked over to the vanity, looked in the mirror, and a big smile appeared on her face. She placed the wild, curly rainbow wig on her head and her smile grew even more. She quickly grabbed the soft red clown nose from the counter and placed it on her own nose to complete the look. *She's no longer a normal little girl, because I have transformed her into a clown all by myself!*

Steve and I took our two little clowns, both of whom I was proud to have created, and headed down the street to obtain as much candy as we could before bedtime. It didn't matter to me that the houses had long driveways. In fact, I was looking forward to walking up each and every one of them, in contrast to using my mobility scooter as I did last year. Steve took Winona's hand and I took Sharon's. The four of us walked up the five steps to the first house. Winona rang the doorbell and when the gentleman answered the door, the girls said, "Trick-or-treat!" in unison. The girls were given two snack-size candy bars. They said "thank you," and then we cut through the yard to the next house. The simple act of walking on thick grass brought me back to my childhood.

* * *

I'm seven, and dressed in a fantastic Indian costume that my mom made just for me. It has everything from the feather on my braided head to a baby doll on my back. It's the perfect costume in my eyes. I have trick-or-treated to about six houses and I'm already exhausted. Every step I take, my knees knock and I insist that I am not going to let myself fall down one more time. The next house we reach has a really long driveway. My friend's father, Dave, suggests to Lonnie that they "just bring Jean's bag of candy up to the house. They'll understand. Take a breather, Jean." Angie and Lonnie gladly run up the long driveway, my bag included, and disappear into the dark of the night. They come back moments later to tell us that they did not secure a treat for me.

"The person who answered the door didn't believe us," Lonnie explains.

"They think we're just trying to get extra candy," Angie says.

Lucky for me, Angie's dad thought to bring the little red wagon with us that evening. They helped me get into it and I continued on my journey to get as much candy as I possibly could.

* * *

I snapped back to reality as my girls and I approached the next house. There was a woman in a festive garage with a game for the girls to play. She explained to them that they needed to spin the wheel to see what she would give them for their treat. Would it be candy, a prize, or cash? As Winona spun the wheel, her body bobbed up and down with anticipation. "Candy it is!" Sharon took her turn and we continued trick-or-treating for the next hour and a half.

To my surprise, Sharon expressed that she was getting tired and wanted to stop. I took her pumpkin to lighten her load. I wanted to keep going. For the first time in my life I realized that trick-or-treating was not a chore. Steve went to get the car as I carried the girls' ten-pound plastic pumpkins to two more houses in disbelief. I couldn't help but ask myself if this was real. *Not only am I carrying these heavy pumpkins a long distance, but I am also creating a new happy memory of Halloween.*

Not every event following my new diagnosis was heartwarming. Less than two years after having the baclofen pump implanted, I faced its removal with a mix of trepidation and joy. *How can it be that after taking baclofen for three decades, I don't need it any longer?*

Neurosurgeon Dr. Gracen informed me that she had done this procedure many times in her career. She reviewed my most recent X-ray and identified precisely which pump-related foreign objects occupied my body. Apparently, there could be some difficulty in removing the tubing that meandered up my back. "This is a common concern," Dr. Gracen explained, as if I should find comfort in this.

"You have a few options. If we remove the tubing, you will need to stay flat on your back for three to ten days, depending on how quickly your body heals. The hole left from the tubing removal needs to mend. If you sit up before the hole closes, cerebrospinal fluid will fill the area, and you'll get a headache like you've never had before. That will land you flat on your back again … so the other option is to remove only the pump—the metal disk. We'd leave the tubing in your spine. There will always be potential for infection if this artificial tubing remains in you, but you will recover from the pump removal much faster."

"Take it all out," I say without hesitation. I have no doubt that God is guiding me in this decision. I'd much rather endure ten days flat on my back now than run the risk of a horrible infection next year, five years from now, or when I'm sixty years old. I confided in Steve and my parents, of course, since this would impact their lives all over again. They agreed, and within a few weeks, I was prepped for another surgery.

I waited in pre-op, hopefully for the last time. *I'll never have to go* to a surgeon again because of my neurological condition, which has sent me to the hospital more times than I care to count. I wasn't sure why, but tears began to sting my eyes. I became a ball of nerves with Steve right by my side.

"What's wrong?" he asked, stepping closer to the bed.

I could only shrug my shoulders, wipe my cheeks, and look away.

"What is it?" Steve asked again.

"I'm scared." For the first time in my life, I was afraid to go under the knife. *I'm chicken. Like other normal people, I'm nervous to be put under with anesthesia ... to put my body in the hands of someone else.*

My past operations were in hopes of gaining some level of mobility, even if it only meant taking steps without holding on to another person. *Now, I'm not gaining anything ... I have everything I always dreamed of having but felt in my heart would never come true. Yet it did! I can walk without help. I can put my kids to bed. I can bake cupcakes for them. And I can drive to see my parents whenever I want. And now, I fear that something will go wrong on this operating table ... it will all be gone before I can truly enjoy it! I'm thirty-four years old and feel like I am living a normal life for the first time. I don't want to mess that up.*

"I'm just nervous is all," I whispered back to Steve.

"You'll do great," he said, patting my back.

* * *

I hit day two of lying flat in bed ... my back muscles throbbing from the lack of movement. More than anything, I wanted to sit up and move to the standard hospital-room chair. Knowing this wasn't an option, I kept my negative thoughts to myself. Yes, this hurt, but it was also temporary. *On the positive side, since I'm not allowed to sit up, I don't feel the piercing pain while moving from bed to chair, which I had when the pump was implanted.* Yes, my cup is always half full.

Flat on my back meant just that, so using a bedpan was out. I hadn't even thought that far ahead when I agreed to the longer recovery option. I had a catheter, which isn't a bad thing. *I'll take it over a bedpan.* However, on this particular hospital stay, the catheter almost caused a major medical setback.

"I feel like I really have to pee," I told the night nurse.

"Well," she explained, "any urine that is in your system will come out into the bag immediately." She checked to make sure that all was connected properly and then added, "It probably just feels like you have to go because your body is a little irritated with the tubing."

After she left the room, I turned to Steve. "I've never felt like I have to pee this badly in my life."

He looked at the empty bag, and inspected the tubing that led from the bag to my vaginal area for kinks. Nothing. We summoned her back, but despite the fact that nothing had gone into the bag for nearly an hour, she insisted that the agonizing discomfort was normal.

In desperation, Steve suggested "Just push the pee out Jean ... maybe there's a small blockage that will clear with a little pressure."

Moments after taking his advice, the bag attached to my bed was nearly full of my urine—1.2 liters! Steve walked to the nurses' station to let them know that this was unacceptable. "After everything she's been through, she could have died from a burst bladder!"

On day three, the neurosurgeon made another visit. Allowing me to look at the horrible cut from the surgeon who had placed the pump, Dr. Gracen explained how she did her best to fix the incision from the pump's placement. It had looked terrible! It reminded me of a short, purple umbilical cord that had been sewn onto my stomach. Not pretty. But when I look at this incision mark today, it is barely visible.

"Have you had a bowel movement yet?" she asked matter-of-factly.

I wanted to lie ... *Yes, of course!* ... I didn't know what her plan of action would be when she heard the truth. Instead, I shook my head, no. She directed the nurses to start some laxatives and I was relieved that a suppository wasn't ordered yet.

"I think it's time to try sitting you up," she smiled at me.

"Are you sure you think the hole is filled?" I asked, clearly questioning her authority. I knew that if I got the bad headache, my bed-bound days would start all over again. My back couldn't take adding additional days to my recovery if they weren't necessary.

As soon as the surgeon walked out of my room, the daytime nurse slowly inclined my hospital bed. "You have been a wonderful patient," she smiled at me.

"Thanks." I had heard this compliment before. The truth is, every time I stayed in the hospital, nurses would tell me I was their easiest patient. I often heard comments like, "Some people think they are the only people we have to care for."

For some reason, I always tried to do whatever I could to show appreciation for everything a nurse would do. Nursing is not a glamorous job, and is often underappreciated. I've always felt it was the nurses who helped the doctors have success with their patients. Their close care for the simple things like helping you go to the bathroom, or even finding the TV remote, minimize the stress to the point where you can do what you are there to do—heal.

I was discharged on day four. As Steve drove me home, I mentally reviewed the past six months. *I'm no longer a spastic diplegia patient. I'm now a dopa-responsive dystonia patient.* I had come so far.

With the pump removed, and finally off all unnecessary meds—with only my new medication, L-dopa, working as the missing link, I was more physical than ever before. At my worst, my daily prescriptions included eleven baclofen pills or the pump's equivalent, one Valium, two metoprolol—typically for high blood pressure, but used to help tame my tremors—and Neurontin for sleep. Feeling drug-free (almost), I didn't want to sit down! *I have spent far too much of my lifetime sitting.* It was finally my chance to get off the couch and really live my life. I let my Facebook Farm die and I began helping Steve with a real garden. I was walking laps inside and outside my house simply because I could. We began eating frozen pizzas more often because I was excited that I could take a pizza out of the oven. My body burned more calories than ever before ... I felt hunger morning, noon, and night! For two weeks, I supplemented my diet with Steve's protein shakes.

Our grocery bill jumped, like we had a teenage boy in our household. Yet, my enthusiasm for food brought new excitement to mealtime. Cooking, cleaning up—who could ever call these "chores"?

Life Is Good
but Someone Is Missing

I can't stop thinking about it. My life has changed so drastically. I can do things now that I never thought possible. If I want to go to the store to shop for clothes, I can do it when and where I want to. I don't have to call up my mother and ask when she is available to go with me, although she is still my favorite shopping buddy. If I want to go for a walk, I can. I don't need to hop on my mobility scooter to see the things in my world that I want to see. My scooter was a helpful tool, but perspective is different from a standing position—especially when the legs that allow this view feel strong and in control. I completed my first-ever ten-mile hike when I returned to Pictured Rocks, one of the most beautiful areas on Lake Superior. In fact, Steve and I retraced the steps of our honeymoon trip, where I had ridden him piggyback for most of our hikes. On this tenth-anniversary return to the same trails, Steve made me walk all of them … and I was elated to do so!

Although I needed hiking shoes for that vacation, I can now splurge from time to time to buy "cute" shoes, including those with a heel! Such a purchase would have been a waste of money in the past. On a visit to Target, not long after my new diagnosis, Mom and I noticed that all of the summer flip-flops and sandals were on sale. I tried on a cute pair just for the heck of it. As I was trying them on, Mom said, "I never thought that I would see the day." They fit perfectly, and actually stayed on my feet with every step I made—so I bought two pair. I was so excited! When we got back to Mom's place, I put them on and walked up and down her driveway. I was so happy, tears filled my eyes and I felt goose bumps from head to toe. As I was walking in them, I could hear Mom telling Sophia, Jack, Sharon, Winona, and Henry that I was never able to wear pretty shoes as a kid.

"She would see them in the store and ask to try them on, but they would never stay on her feet," Mom explained to her little listeners. I don't know if the kids understood why this was such a milestone for me, but I vow I will never forget that Target shoe-shopping day as long as I live.

* * *

For the first time in my life, I could volunteer at my daughter's school and for extracurricular activities. I was planning the Halloween party for Winona's third-grade class. I also began teaching her religious education class, and became the co-leader of her Brownie troop. I began volunteering in Sharon's class too. Every Friday morning I went to listen to children in her class read to me.

One night, I drove Sharon to Daisies, then the very next evening I was picking the girls up at school and taking Winona to Brownies. In past years, my mom had to drive us everywhere in the evening because I was too spastic by that time of day. Life seemed incredibly easy!

So, why was I spending so much of each day wondering about having another child? *I have two healthy, beautiful daughters that I wouldn't trade for the world. Why do I think I need three?* Growing them in my disabled body was by far the hardest thing that I had ever done in my life. The spasms were so strong that I couldn't get regular sleep or keep food down. I could barely walk or write with a pen. I knew that I was going to have two children no matter how difficult it was for me to carry each of them. Yet while pregnant with Sharon, I survived under the premise that *never in a million years will I have another child.* I would joke with my mom, "If I ever get pregnant

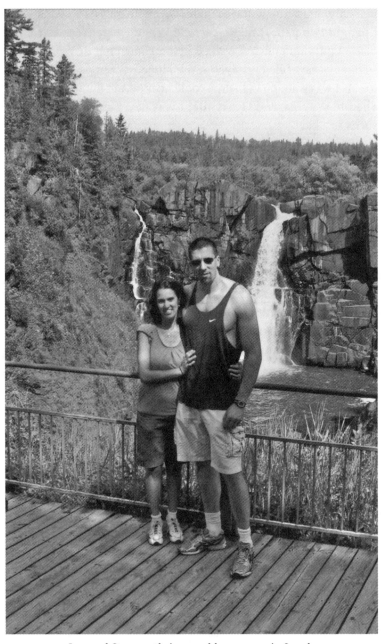

Jean and Steve on their second honeymoon in Canada

again, my first call will be to the state hospital to come lock me up." I knew that I could only do it twice … to keep Winona from being an only child.

I recalled my argument with the nurse at that prenatal appointment for Sharon when I wanted my tubes tied. I'll never forget her saying, "You can't make a decision about that while you are feeling like this." I knew in my heart two children were enough to complete our family. So, why did the thought of another child make my heart so heavy?

I don't know what to do. My girls are eight and six. If we conceived a child today, Winona and Sharon will be nine and seven when the baby comes into the world. That is such a big gap in their ages. A third child would forever change the dynamic of our family. It would make going on a family vacation more work. We would have to worry about naps, bottles, and diapers again. As it is now, Steve doesn't like to stop the car to let one of us pee at the gas station. He's on a mission to get there, wherever our destination. I could only imagine how a baby would change all of this.

I will call this period in my life my Baby Obsession. Throughout this inner struggle, which lasted weeks—maybe months—Steve was gone at work much of the day. He had a routine of stopping at the gym on his way home, so he and the girls were lucky if they saw one another on a school night. If he made it home before their bedtimes, I often had a household task for him to complete.

There are so many things that need to get done around the condo, it's not even funny. We've been here for six months and the shower curtain isn't up in the girls' bathroom. We don't have any pictures on the wall, and the guest room is filled with bins that still need to be unpacked. How can I possibly consider bringing another child into this very busy and complicated home?

Yet, I wanted to know what it was like to stand and place my calm hands on a swelling baby belly without my shaking, rigid arms pulling away. I wanted to actually hold a baby in those moments after an exhausting delivery. I wanted to stand and rock my child to sleep in my arms, while rubbing the smooth soft skin of her head to my cheek. I wanted my baby to take her first steps with me standing right behind, holding her hands. *I could bring her into preschool, instead of having to wait for the teacher to come out to the car to get her. I* imagined bending over to pick her up off the floor … holding her at the stove while I stirred dinner. These were all things that most mothers had the privilege of doing, that—even after two babies—I had yet to experience. *I'm just not sure that these are reasons enough to bring another child into the world.*

I did know this. I would be a great mom to this next child. I just wasn't sure if it would be fair to the rest of the family. These thoughts—my Baby Obsession—monopolized my daydreams. And then I began sharing some of it with the girls. Winona and Sharon of course wanted me to have another baby … *but I know they don't understand how much work a baby is. I have two healthy, happy girls. Now I just need to decide if there should be one more.*

My Baby Obsession was becoming a problem. This perpetual internal dialogue of baby-weighing reasons to give birth just one more time played like a broken record in my mind. I desperately wanted to feel a fetus roll around in my stomach … to feel that first flutter. I obsessed over watching her stretch while she slept and then imagined picking her up with ease when she woke. *Would she look like me or Steve? How would Sharon and Winona be as older sisters? It would turn this family upside down … How can I do that to them?*

But, I would be able to carry the car seat for the first time—with the baby in it—out to the car. I'm a mother of two beautiful daughters and I have never carried a baby car seat into the house. I had pushed a baby in a stroller. I had fed both the girls and changed their diapers. *If I could do a lot of that when I was immobile, it would be much easier now, right? … To do this and so much more.* There wasn't a moment's rest from my Baby Obsession of pros and cons.

Stop. This is a selfish want for someone who has just been given so many gifts in life. I began blocking the whole thing out of my mind. How could I ignore that our family was the perfect size? Many things in life are made for a family of four. *Let's see all the things I can list that are meant for the perfect-sized Abbott family: a hotel room, our car, our cabin, a booth at a restaurant …* I tried my best to cherish what we already had, and stop imagining what we were missing.

But at night, my challenge of rejecting this new baby became impossible. I lost sleep while I searched for names—boys as well as girls—and tried to predict what Steve would think if he knew how obsessed I was. *I can't talk to him about this. At least not yet. I know his answer—he would love to have another baby.* The topic had come up on our anniversary tour of Lake Superior. I couldn't share any of this with Steve until I was 100 percent certain that I would go ahead with having number three. I couldn't get his hopes up and then deflate them. I knew that if I even hinted to Steve, it meant the decision had been made. *God, please guide me in yet another important decision.*

Every possible pregnancy topic invaded my thoughts—even some that scared me far more than hauling a Pack and Play on vacation. *I don't know if I can take the risk of having a child with Down syndrome. We are blessed with two healthy girls who have the potential to be as independent as they want to be some day. To us, they are perfect!* By now, I was pushing thirty-five—an age where the odds are 1 in 400 of having a Down syndrome baby.

All that I had been through, all that God had given me since that visit to Courage Center ... I had to be completely honest with myself. *I don't want to face the struggles of a disabled child. It would be so hard.*

Ironic, I know. Who better equipped to raise a child with Down syndrome, or any kind of disability, than a mother who had lived it? But my inner thoughts were frank and honest. I had endured so much, been given the miracle of mobility—*why would I mess with this?*

The idea of having a boy scared me also. Little boys are so full of energy. They get into everything ... cause messes and break things. They don't seem to have any fear. They are willing to try anything, at least once. You parents of boys have permission to chuckle at me ... as if gender should be feared like an illness ... or has anything to do with free-spirited kids who get into things we never saw coming. But my fear of having a boy was present nonetheless, and it sparred with my relentless Baby Obsession. Soon, my inner dialogue got busy designing the perfect infant boy.

He would be so handsome, especially if he looks like Steve. I'm sure he would be tall ... with Steve's love for the game, maybe he'd be a great bas-

ketball player. But my dreams turned to worries as I weighed all of the things that could go wrong. My parents found out firsthand that there are no guarantees when having a child. They had not bargained for all the challenges I brought to their lives. *Can we take a chance that our lives might change forever if something goes wrong ... and so soon after being gifted a miracle?*

While my Baby Obsession invaded my every thought, random pregnancy ads captured my attention. My favorite ... a broad, unscientific quiz on Facebook. *Now this simplifies life's direst decisions!* A fast, fortune-telling teaser promised to foreshadow something significant for 2011. My survey results? I would a. become pregnant or b. have a baby. *What a range of possibilities!* Although I never even answered one question about childbirth, the outcome was unequivocally baby-stacked. *That's Facebook for you.* I decided to avoid the quiz entitled, "When will you die?" *It will likely have me dying while giving birth this year.* My morbid sense of humor kicked in at times like this.

While my inner debate raged on, I recalled how sick I was while pregnant with the girls. *I threw up a lot ... I think I started every morning with my cereal coming up. Nine months of that ... times two!* Then, the voice of reason would counter with something like ... *I hear they have a shot for that now. And actually, much of my nausea was probably due to medication withdrawal.* As my two-way inner monologues continued, I began to think my new diagnosis came with schizophrenia.

Just when I recalled enough of the miserable memories of pregnancy, I would find a rational way to handle things. But of course, there were always the "traditional" female fears ...

I'm scared that I will gain weight! Just when I am back into a size eight jeans ... that's the same size I wore in college. In fact, I weigh the same as I did then. If I go through another pregnancy who's to say that I won't gain lots of weight and never take it off ... at this age, that's possible.

It had taken me several years to lose my baby weight from Sharon. I guess it didn't help that I couldn't walk on my own at that time ... I didn't exactly have a method to exercise the weight away back then.

Of all my baby misgivings, my most logical reason to end the urge to procreate once more was actually a legitimate medical concern. Extremely loathsome and incredibly painful … I had just recovered from a hemorrhoidectomy. Two months after the procedure, I was finally feeling the cure for a vascular cluster that is quite common for those who sit too much. A lack of mobility during the final years of my misdiagnosis compounded a problem that might recur if I pushed the third-baby idea. I had to confront the fact that if I developed another hemorrhoid problem, I would *not* opt for surgery again. I might let the memory of labor pains fade … but an unbearable recovery like that would never be forgotten.

Someone, just tell me what to do! Are you listening, God?

After consulting my friends, and stalking almost every infant and toddler I encountered that summer, the debate truly came down to one question: *Am I too old? If I get pregnant now, at thirty-five, I'll be thirty-six when I have the kid. I'll be forty-one when he/she gets on the bus to go to kindergarten and fifty-two when he/she gets a driver's license. At fifty-four, Steve and I will be watching our last child walk across the stage to receive a high school diploma, and at fifty-eight or fifty-nine we'll hopefully see our last one get his undergraduate degree. Forget grandchildren … I'll be too old and tired for that!*

Finally, I left the whole debate to the decision-maker's oldest technique … the flip of a coin. In jest one day, I grabbed a quarter … *heads I'll have a baby and tails I won't.* The result … *Heads! That's it. I guess I'll need a baby shower! The only thing I have left from the girls is a Pack and Play.*

* * *

April 30, 2011: I caught myself crying one night while watching *Grey's Anatomy* … a baby episode, of course. *I want a baby and no matter how many times I talk myself out of it, I wake up the next morning dreaming of holding a new life.*

Memories of being home alone with our girls while Steve worked through bedtimes came racing back to me. It never felt right … never good enough … to lay my baby on the floor, look into her eyes and think to myself, *you deserve to sleep in a crib.* But I would kiss her cheek, whether it was Winona or Sharon, turn out the light, and stumble back to my bedroom to fight the feeling that I was a horrible mother ... *I'm probably the only mother in America who leaves her child on the floor for the night.*

Deep in my heart, I always knew that I was doing the right thing. *They were safer* ... rather than risk carrying each of them on a shaky walk from the living room to their cribs. My mom always told me they were safe. Steve did too. But I still fought the feeling that I was failing them. *I would love to carry my baby without the fear that I could hurt him/her in some way.*

As the *Grey's Anatomy* credits scrolled by that night, I concluded there was no easy answer. I thought again of the way my friend Diana said it: "You will never regret having another baby, but you may regret not having one." *She is absolutely right.*

My Baby Obsession took over during the dark hours of sleeplessness that night. *I'm going to the clinic tomorrow to have my IUD taken out.* Yet, I woke the next morning as I always did ... with a changed mindset. *Why is this? How can I ever follow through with baby number three if I chicken out with the start of a new day? I'll have to count on the good Lord to help guide me again. Please, I need what feels like another miracle, God!*

* * *

October 26, 2011: I was nine weeks pregnant and very excited. I felt sick all day, but found nausea so much easier to tolerate than the last two pregnancies. I could walk, use my arms, make my own meals, and drive. *This is going to be so much easier ... as long as there are no unexpected complications.*

I finally found the courage to have my IUD taken out early that summer. I think I have made it clear—this was not a decision I took lightly! Regardless of the minor inconveniences so far, I am very happy with this decision, and excited for the May due date so we can greet this baby for the first time.

When we told the girls that I was going to have a baby, they seemed shocked, but happy at the same time. We were on our way

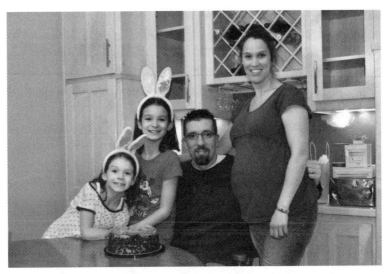

Sharon, Winona, Steve, Jean, and baby-to-be on Steve's birthday

to my OB sonogram appointment, and decided they should come along to see the baby on the monitor. They seemed to enjoy this! The baby was only the size of Steve's thumbnail. The tech told the girls that we might even be able to see the baby move. On cue, the baby began to dance on the screen. "It looks like a teddy bear," I said, and they all agreed.

This baby is loved and it doesn't even have limbs yet. I prayed every day that this baby would be healthy, and I would have the strength to do what I needed to do to bring him or her into the world.

When we got home from the appointment, Steve and I decided to use the sonogram printout to tell his family and mine the good news. The next day, we made our way to Bennigan's to meet my parents. "We should get together so Steve can tell you about his new job," I had said on the phone. They didn't know that we had two big news items to share.

At the restaurant, Steve began explaining that in his new position, he would be making a heart valve. He then handed my parents the photo of the baby. They both stared in silence. My nerves began to signal to me … maybe this wasn't the best way to communicate this news. *What if they think we're crazy? What if I'm bringing more worry to them?* Finally, my dad said, "This looks like a baby."

Ha! The silence is explained. What a relief!

"It is a baby. We're having a baby, Dad. Can you believe it? Grandpa again!"

Mom and Dad were both so excited. And I think I saw tears in Dad's eyes while Mom cheered over the good news. I don't think I'll ever forget that moment.

After hugs from both, I asked them if they were surprised. I was stunned when my mom said, "Not really." She had been wondering if we would have another one and said, "I almost asked you a couple weeks ago."

"I was afraid to tell you—I thought you and Dad would think we were crazy!"

After lunch we went to Tom's to tell him the news. He seemed happy, but I couldn't help think he was glad it wasn't him … which made me chuckle to myself.

On Sunday we went to my parents since Mike and Cathy were returning from a camping trip. We forgot the picture, so telling them would have to be different. I said to Mike, "We've got some really good news. Steve got a job."

Mike said, "Oh, that's great! … I thought maybe you were going to tell me baby number three was on the way."

"Well, that too," I said.

"What? You're kidding!" Mike replied. "That's great. He jumped up and gave me a hug. I think that's when it hit Cathy. They were both very happy for us.

* * *

On May 20, I was blessed with a beautiful, healthy baby boy. We named him John Stephen. I always find it so amazing how fast you can love another human being. I'm marveling at how much easier it all happened this time around.

Like my daughters, baby John is a really good baby. He eats well and sleeps well. Because my mobility is so much better than it was when my girls were born, I find true enjoyment feeding this little guy at 3:00 A.M. My legs can walk me to the kitchen to make his bottle and my hands allow me to easily change his dirty diapers. It was so challenging taking care of the girls. I could do it all, but it would take me so much longer to snap up their sleepers and fasten their diapers.

I may have three children now, but today was the first day that I ever gave an infant a bath. Steve always took care of that for me in the past. Even though John cried the whole time, I loved *every* second of it and can't imagine ever forgetting that I did it on my own.

My life is very busy taking care of two girls, ages ten and eight, and my one-week-old son, but I can honestly say that I have never been this happy. I have everything I could ever want: a great husband, three healthy kids, and a safe place we call home. I wouldn't want to trade places with anyone else in the world, and I thank God for all the wonderful gifts He has given me.

33 AD:
My Life "After Diagnosis"

Dear friends and family,

I have life-changing information that I am excited to share with all of you who have supported me and my family since I was a young child.

On Good Friday, I went to see a new neurologist, who came to a shocking conclusion—I was misdiagnosed as a child. I have DRD (dopa-responsive dystonia), not spastic diplegia. DRD is a neurological disorder that is characterized by abnormal muscle tone that responds extremely well to a drug that increases levels of the neurotransmitter dopamine. The critical piece of the puzzle was the fact that my condition is best immediately after I wake up. It turns out that dopamine production is highest while you sleep.

She informed me that if this diagnosis was correct I would be able to do normal activities without thinking about it. I have to admit that I was skeptical and had my doubts. In fact, I wasn't even going to start taking the medication the day of the appointment. I was just going to wait until the next day. My optimistic husband, Steve, urged me to start right away. I'm pleased to say that I noticed a remarkable change in my physical limitations immediately. Every day I'm able to do several new things that I never thought possible. I'm enjoying all of the little things in life. Today I made cupcakes for the first time ever without help!

I am grateful for the life that the good Lord has given me. I had a childhood that I wouldn't change for a minute. I wouldn't be the person who I am today without the life experiences I had due to my physical limitations. We don't know for sure what the future holds for me, but I think it looks pretty darned good.

Jean

As long as I can remember, I always told myself that "everything happens for a reason." This is not something that I heard from my parents. It was not a phrase I picked up on in CCD or the study of Ecclesiastes 3: "To everything there is a season, and a time to every purpose under Heaven ... He hath made everything beautiful in His time ... " That connection clicked much later in life ... only after my new diagnosis and while reflecting on things for this book. Rather, this was a simple saying I told myself, and sometimes others, as a mantra to accept my circumstances and move forward.

Life had always been challenging for me. Whether it was dealing with a classmate for making fun of my walk, or frustration when I couldn't do something that was physically easy for others, I knew in my heart that God had made me this way for a reason.

In my childhood religious education, we all learned early on that "God doesn't make mistakes." Having been taught this, I assumed that since I was born with a muscle disorder and all the limitations that come with disability, God apparently wanted me like this. *He must want others to see my positive attitude and maybe take a look at themselves ... to see if they are making the most out of the life that He has given them.* I don't want to sound arrogant, like I was the chosen one. That's not how I feel, nor was I always accepting of my physical limitations. But the thought of being picked by God to share a message to others in their time on Earth—well, this helped me accept my circumstances ... and deep down I know it's the truth. I know that God provides opportunities for all of us to shine if we just see our situation in the right light.

I also grew up being told that God will never give us more than we can handle. This phrase actually scares me a little bit. Having to deal with my limitations—both my hand dexterity and my uncooperative legs—I had to work harder to get the same outcome as the person standing next to me. Most of my peers didn't enter the high school cafeteria fearing that if they dropped their lunch tray on the floor, everyone would turn, look, and wonder, *What's wrong with that girl?* Although it never happened, the concern crossed my mind daily, especially those times when I could barely put one foot in front of the other. I often thought, *Why does God think I can handle so much?*

My new diagnosis, however, provided a new slant on this saying. Knowing that God doesn't give us more than we can handle scared me. I feared things pending for which God viewed me as too weak to handle in my current physical state. *What's so bad that God knows I won't be able to handle it as a disabled mom?* This makes me rather sad, and afraid to wonder, *What does my future hold that is so horrible? Will my kids be involved? Will it be Steve, my rock? Will he need a stronger me? Apparently, God thinks I must be more able-bodied to endure these things.* And then I think, *Perhaps God believes it's simply time for a new purpose … Jean Abbott has endured enough.* Maybe my physical struggles have set the groundwork for a different message to share.

Regardless of the changes in my life, I have and always will believe that God made me different so I can show people that there is so much in life to be grateful for. Those who knew me as a child watched me go to public school and not take the short bus. Both my peers and adults around me saw that I earned good grades and spoke well with and of others. People watched me go off to college even after my career counselor, who should have been my biggest advocate, told me that I should stay at home and go to the community college. I can't deny that others' doubts influenced me at times … I thought about her advice for a couple days and I doubted my abilities to attend Winona State. Yet, my parents told me that if I wanted to go to college, I should go ahead and do it. They reminded me that both my brothers' guidance counselors told them the same thing: they would struggle or fail in college. When I look back at that time in my life, I know I was sad and had self-doubts because of my counselor's words … and now, I get angry with that woman. Had I listened to her, I wouldn't have met my husband or had my beautiful daughters. Yet, this probably planted a defense in my mind that I truly needed. Her words—her doubts—put me on my guard to succeed at college. I had something to prove, even if, in the end, her opinion meant nothing to me. That initial motivation surely helped me. *Everything happens for a reason.*

Whenever I tell someone who didn't know me before my new diagnosis that I used to be disabled … that I had many limitations … that I endured some painful procedures growing up … they almost always ask, "Does it make you angry that it took doctors so long to figure out your correct diagnosis?" My answer is almost always the same: "No. If I had grown up with my new medication I would have probably gone to a different college. I wouldn't have met my husband. I wouldn't have had the outlook on life that I have today. I might have taken my parents and all of their sacrifices for granted. My struggle was a gift … and I am blessed to see the before and after of it. All of the experiences I had along the way have made me the person I am today … and I like me."

If I had been a "normal" kid, my life would have been completely different. For one thing, I would have surely faced peer pressure. I was never part of the popular crowd, so I never went to parties where there may have been pressure to try drugs or alcohol. When I was in high school, the guys were not interested in me. Since I never went on a date in high school, I didn't deal with a guy trying to pressure me into having sex at a young age. I would like to think that my parents taught me well and that I would have exercised the morals and self-esteem to tell someone "No," but the fact of the matter is that it was a relief to not have to deal with that in the first place … even if I thought I'd die a virgin. Who knows, maybe I would have gotten pregnant in high school … had five kids by now … been living in a run-down neighborhood because I never went to college. I really don't know. What I do know is that God had a plan for me. And God has a plan for others who find themselves in the circumstances that I dodged due to my disability. Yet, it would be wrong for me to claim that my life was worse than those who must face difficult decisions at a very young age. In many ways, my disability protected me. How can I be angry about this?

I will always be grateful for the life that I was given. Things could have been very different for me if God's plan had been different. I could have had a mental disability rather than a physical one. I think that would have been much more challenging because I believe that the world is less accepting and understanding of people with internal disabilities … the kind that are invisible to others. I think the most difficult thing to try to live with would be depression. For the most part, I was a really happy kid. I had lots of friends and was almost always rushing (in my own way) out the door to do things. I never sat around feeling sorry for myself. I wasn't about to waste my time with that. Yet, my baclofen-pump episode gave me a taste of life in decline. I had my down days—compounded by medications—and didn't know if they were temporary. I struggled and felt depressed just long enough to know that this must be a horrific struggle for those with chronic depression and other mental illnesses. What turned out temporary for me has given me a level of empathy for others that I hope I never forget.

So, in the spring of my thirty-third year, God must have thought that I'd had enough. It was time to make me whole. God knew that I would show and tell the world that I could now physically do whatever I wanted … and I can't help notice that most of these things are the daily chores in life that others dread. There are all kinds of things out there that most Americans hate to do, but I love, because I could never do them in the past.

Things I Enjoy that Others Dislike:
- putting clean sheets on a bed
- cooking meals
- driving the kids to all of their activities
- braiding my daughters' hair
- changing my baby into his PJs for the night
- walking door-to-door for the kids' fundraisers
- volunteering at school
- grocery shopping (I don't know anyone who enjoys grocery shopping.)

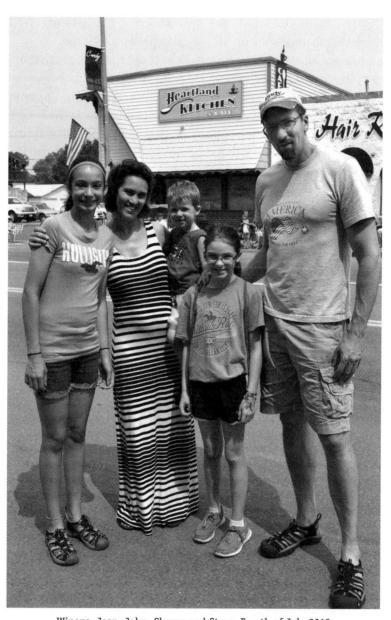

Winona, Jean, John, Sharon and Steve, Fourth of July 2015

My friends and family see me embracing these things and I think that their outlook on life has changed a little bit too.

I hope I have taught people, or at least reminded them, that life is a gift. You have the choice to make the most out of it or waste it. The little things in life matter the most. My kids love that I can put them to bed at night. I couldn't always do that before. I vow always to remember that when I was at a real low in my life, Winona was putting me to bed. I would get home from work, I would use the bathroom with Winona's help, and she would help me get into my pajamas. She was only five years old. Those picnic nights of peanut butter and jelly sandwiches on a bath towel in my bedroom worked at the time. The three of us, hanging out together, sharing a movie and a meal, precious hours of family time that so many people never have with their children today. When I think of kids going off to their own bedrooms, parents too busy to even read them a book, I am grateful for the slower pace I had with Winona and Sharon during those early years. Yet, now when life's responsibilities call me into action, I embrace the opportunity to be busy and hop to so many things I couldn't even attempt back then.

I think God wanted me to be physically disabled as a young mom so my girls could see exactly what it's like to live with physical limitations. They will be able to teach their generation not to take things for granted. I really think this is the reason God waited so long to introduce me to Dr. Williams and Dr. Griffith.

I'm no longer the Rainy Day Friend … I hope I'm the rain-or-shine friend, especially to those who believed in me—who loved me even with all of my difficulties … even when I caused their own heartache. When Mom and I talked recently about this book, I reminded her that I chose *her* words for the name of my blog. She smiled. And that's when it dawned on me. My disability was part of my mom's thoughts every single day … morning, noon, and night. As I selfishly dwelled on not being able to run outside with my friends, she worried about things like, *Will Jeanie ever live a normal life? Will she go away to college … will my daughter marry or have children?* She was consumed with worry over me, much like my Baby

Obsession, but the only difference was that my thoughts were about something that could be absolutely wonderful, while her thoughts were filled with one *what if* after another.

* * *

There is always a reason. God doesn't make mistakes. I trust in His judgment, and hope others can see their own struggles with new eyes.

Epilogue

SO MUCH HAS HAPPENED SINCE THE DISCOVERY OF MY NEW diagnosis. Besides this book and my family changes, I have discovered the power of sharing via social-networking avenues like Facebook, Happify.com, and my own blog, JeanAbbott.com. I hope that readers will take the time to check in on my wonderfully new life, not only for the pleasure of showing how different things are for me, but because we never know who we may help via our own stories, our own struggles, and our own accomplishments.

Just in the short time I have been blogging, I have connected with twenty people who have directly benefitted from asking their doctors more questions, or seeking second opinions regarding their own misunderstood diagnoses. One mom contacted me to let me know that because of my story she took her daughter in to try L-dopa. When her physician said "no" to the new medication, she went to a different doctor who did prescribe her daughter the "miracle drug." I was so pleased to hear that in a short time her daughter was able to walk without her crutches. Hearing stories like hers makes everything I went through worth it. I have always felt joy in helping others, but this brings it to a whole new level.

Here are a few of my blog entries that will hopefully inspire readers to consider the power of sharing, and the miracles that can happen when we follow someone else's journey.

* * *

First Dance

June 5, 2011

Yesterday was by far one of the best days of my life. I attended my first wedding since my new diagnosis. Everything from the wedding to the reception brought me tears of joy.

When the reception began and the DJ started the music, I was immediately brought to my feet by my dad pulling me to the dance floor. I eagerly followed his lead and we were dancing to the upbeat music. I have to admit, I felt a little awkward. I had no idea how to dance and my sense of rhythm was anything but graceful. It really didn't matter though. All I really cared about was that I was having fun with my dad. We smiled at one another and I can't help but think how happy he looked to see me up and dancing with him.

Last night I learned that I *love* to dance. As I said earlier, I had no idea what I was doing, but I didn't care. There was just something about bopping around the dance floor with my daughters, husband, nieces, nephews, cousins, sisters-in-law, brothers, and parents. We had a blast dancing to everything from Kid Rock to the Chicken Dance. I even did the Conga!

I patiently waited all evening for a slow song. It was really important to me that I have the father/daughter dance that I was unable to do at my own wedding nearly eleven years ago. When American Soldier began playing, I knew I had to get my dad out on the dance floor. He gladly accepted my request. Again, I didn't know what I was doing and my dad showed me how to follow his lead, something that I was unable to learn from him years earlier. As I got the hang of slow dancing, I felt it was necessary to tell him all things that I never got to say on the dance floor at my own wedding. He reminded me that everything always works itself out in the end and he was right. By the end of the song, we both had tears in our eyes and unexpectedly I found myself giving my dad a hug and telling him that I love him.

This is clearly a wedding that I will never forget. Last night I was given the gift of dancing with my family; a gift that I will never take for granted.

* * *

Huge Accomplishment

May 9, 2012

What an evening. My Martial Arts instructor came over tonight so he could work with me on my kicks. Even though I could have this baby any day now, I stretched and prepared for the lesson. He patiently reviewed several different kicks with me and I did each one a few times. I was really surprised how well it was going since my balance has been off during this last month of pregnancy.

When we were all done going through the kicks, he left the room momentary and returned with Steve and my girls behind him. I could see that Sharon was holding something behind her back and was stunned to see her holding a white-and-gold striped belt that was meant to replace the white belt that I have been wearing for over a year.

My instructor then handed me the official certificate that stated I have earned the new belt. I couldn't help but smile and look at my mom sitting on the couch and say, "I bet you never thought you'd see me do this."

Then my instructor handed me a red star patch (goal patch) and had Steve read yet another certificate. As he read it, I could feel the tears in my eyes and could see my father tearing up as well. I don't think anyone in the room ever thought they'd see the day that I would accomplish something in a sport. Certainly not me. This certificate says the following:

> This Goal Star Award is Hereby Presented to:
> Jean Abbott
> Your Indomitable Spirit, Perseverance, Self Control, and unwavering Integrity is an inspiration to everyone. To have overcome what you have, without spite of others, and always looking ahead to new challenges with the perseverance to conquer what stands in your way, you inspire others to be better than what they are and show them a path to that goal.

I think that these are some of the nicest words ever said about me. The fact of the matter is, I could not have accomplished this goal without my instructor or my family. With that all being said, I think it's time for this baby to be born!

* * *

Miracle in the Badlands
August 27, 2012

This past weekend, I was fortunate to have the opportunity to hike in The Badlands. Using my hiking poles, I was able to walk independently with Steve and the girls. As the sun beat on my face and the silence rang in my ears, all I could do was thank God for the wonderful gift He had placed before me. I couldn't keep the tears from my eyes and felt that I had to tell my girls how lucky we were. Not only were we able to look at God's beautiful work, but we were also blessed to be right in the heart of it, together as a family.

There were several times on this walk that I wasn't sure if I could make it all the way to the end of the trail. Every time I found myself up really high on a rock or on a narrow path, Steve assured me that I could do it. Every step of the way, I could tell that he was proud to be with me on this exciting experience. I desperately needed his support and because of it, I was able to make it to what felt like the end of the earth.

* * *

Cooking with DRD
June 25, 2013

Even though I have always tried to keep a positive attitude, I hated to cook! In the past, it would take me double to triple the time to make a classic Minnesota hotdish (a can of creamed soup, meat, and noodles). Plus, the end result wasn't as good as what most people could make. Mine would often be overcooked and dry. In fact, Sharon would use ketchup at nearly every meal to mask the taste. Through the years of struggling to cook I became very unsure of my abilities and doubted myself a great deal. Therefore, we ate frozen lasagna and other entrees weekly.

One year ago, I decided that enough was enough and I was going to teach myself how to cook! At first, I wouldn't change a single thing about any recipe that I found online, fearing that if I did it would turn out terribly. In the beginning, I'd often call my parents or e-mail Steve at work with questions such as, "How do I know when the pork chops are done?" or "Why should I use fresh garlic over powdered garlic?" It's been quite the journey. My cooking has improved a great deal and I even feel comfortable cooking for those who are not in my family.

After I try making a new recipe, I often feel proud of myself. In fact, yesterday I made two loaves of white bread. After three hours of prep and baking, I pulled the pans out of the oven and all but jumped up and down with gratitude because it looked just like it was supposed to. The kids and I took a taste and their expressions told me that I exceeded their expectations. I think the girls were just as happy as I was that I succeeded in my baking. I can't believe how far I have come in this last year and am so excited to continue creating more delicious meals for my family, without it feeling like such a chore.

* * *

Thankful Beyond Words
June 4, 2013

Once again, I was overcome with so much joy. My niece Mikaela chose me to be her sponsor for her Confirmation. I met up with her and the rest of my family at the Cathedral of St. Paul. The beauty of the church alone is enough to stir up emotion in me, but knowing I had the ability to walk around among the hundreds of people and be a part of Mikaela's Confirmation brought tears to my eyes.

Fourteen years ago, I went to Mikaela's baptism. I had difficulty standing and sat for most of the day. As I stood behind her in the long line waiting for her turn to be confirmed last night, many thoughts swam through my head: *How did she grow up so fast? How can I be standing here in this long line independently? I'm wearing sandals and I'm not worried that I'll walk right out of them (or fall).* And then I felt the presence of God as a bright light shone above me. All I could do is pray for Mikaela and give thanks for the life He has given me.

Book Club Questions

1. What do you feel the purpose of this book was? Do you think the author reached that goal?
2. What do you feel the author left out of this book? What lesson do you feel could be taken from reading this book? How did it change your perspective on life?
3. How does having a disabled child change the dynamics in a family? Do you think the author's parents and siblings are angry that she went so many years misdiagnosed?
4. What do you think Steve's parents thought when he told them he was going to marry a disabled girl? Would you encourage or discourage a relationship like this?
5. Was Jean a good mother even though she was disabled? Do you think she was selfish in having children? Should she have stopped after the first child?
6. Was Jean's high school counselor right in discouraging her from going away to college? How would you have handled that situation?
7. How did Jean's positive attitude help her get through her struggles? How would you have reacted during some of those difficult times (the lady in the parking lot who thought she was drunk, the co-worker who suggested she terminate her pregnancy, the boss who wanted to cut her pay, etc.)?
8. How have things changed for disabled people since Jean was growing up in the 1980s?

9. If you were Jean, would you have thought about a lawsuit against her doctors?

10. Who were the heroes in Jean's story?

11. How does Jean's story encourage everyone, not just disabled people?

12. Do you consider Jean's correct diagnosis a medical miracle or a miracle from a higher power?

13. Jean worked hard to overcome many obstacles in life; do you think most people would have handled her situation differently?

14. If you could tell Jean anything, what would it be?

15. Do you think Jean's parents were wrong in not putting her in a wheelchair at an earlier age? Do you think her life would have been easier?

16. Jean's mom said that "there is someone for everyone." Do you think that is true or do you think she was giving her false hope?

best of your situation. . . . the seniors hung on to every word you spoke. Standing ovations are rare at the Senior Center, so when the audience jumped to their feet at the conclusion of your presentation, it was true confirmation that you pulled at their heartstrings and touched them with your story . . ."

—Kris N., Coon Rapids Senior Center, Coon Rapids, MN

". . . Jean's attitude of **perseverance mixed with gratitude** is outstanding. Her story will reach individuals who can be properly diagnosed as well as people learning resiliency!"

—Nancy D., Winona, MN

More praise from those inspired by Jean's story:

"TheMighty.com has published 5,000 stories that have been read by 75 million people, and the single most powerful one is Jean Abbott's. Her story has literally changed people's lives. **What's remarkable about Jean is not her condition, but her attitude and approach to it.** Everyone facing a challenging health situation will gain so much from her words."

—Mike Porath, Founder/CEO, TheMighty.com

"Because of you, my son has also been diagnosed with DRD and is now on the meds he needs. I repeat, 'because of you,' because I want you to know that I am so thankful to you, you are helping so many people in such a big way, being **instrumental in changing their lives for the better . . .**"

—Melinda E., Las Vegas, NV

". . . I *love* your outlook on life and your past. Truly an inspiration. **We can all look to your example for when life hands us a 'raw deal,'** which apparently, because of your optimism, you actually see as a blessing . . ."

—Kerry P., Frisco, TX

". . . You were [an] inspirational and motivational [speaker]—giving everyone in the room a life lesson on how to **always make the**